CHRISTIAN THEOLOGY AND MEDICAL ETHICS

Theology and Medicine

VOLUME 7

Managing Editor

Earl E. Shelp, *The Foundation for Interfaith Research & Ministry, Houston, Texas*

Editorial Board

James F. Childress, *Department of Religious Studies, University of Virginia, Charlottesville, Virginia*

Margaret A. Farley, *The Divinity School, Yale University, New Haven, Connecticut*

Ronald M. Green, *Department of Religion, Dartmouth College, Hanover, New Hampshire*

Stanley Hauerwas, *The Divinity School, Duke University, Durham, North Carolina*

Richard A. McCormick, S.J., *Department of Theology, University of Notre Dame, Notre Dame, Indiana*

Wayne Proudfoot, *Department of Religion, Columbia University, New York*

The titles published in this series are listed at the end of this volume.

CHRISTIAN THEOLOGY AND MEDICAL ETHICS

Four Contemporary Approaches

by

JAMES B. TUBBS, JR.

*University of Detroit Mercy,
Detroit, MI, USA*

KLUWER ACADEMIC PUBLISHERS
DORDRECHT / BOSTON / LONDON

Library of Congress Cataloging-in-Publication Data

```
Tubbs, James B.
   Christian theology and medical ethics : four contemporary
approaches / by James B. Tubbs, Jr.
      p.    cm.  -- (Theology and medicine ; v. 7)
   Includes index.
   ISBN 0-7923-3657-7 (alk. paper)
   1. Medical ethics--Religious aspects--Christianity. 2. Christian
ethics--History--20th century.   I. Title.   II. Series.
R725.56.T83  1996
174'.2--dc20                                                 95-31705
```

ISBN 0-7923-3657-7

Published by Kluwer Academic Publishers,
P.O. Box 17, 3300 AA Dordrecht, The Netherlands.

Kluwer Academic Publishers incorporates
the publishing programmes of
D. Reidel, Martinus Nijhoff, Dr W. Junk and MTP Press.

Sold and distributed in the U.S.A. and Canada
by Kluwer Academic Publishers,
101 Philip Drive, Norwell, MA 02061, U.S.A.

In all other countries, sold and distributed
by Kluwer Academic Publishers Group,
P.O. Box 322, 3300 AH Dordrecht, The Netherlands.

Printed on acid-free paper

All Rights Reserved
© 1996 Kluwer Academic Publishers
No part of the material protected by this copyright notice may be reproduced or
utilized in any form or by any means, electronic or mechanical,
including photocopying, recording or by any information storage and
retrieval system, without written permission from
the copyright owner.

Printed in the Netherlands

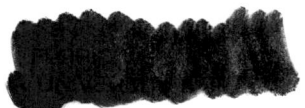

To Leonora C. Tubbs and James B. Tubbs

TABLE OF CONTENTS

Acknowledgements	ix
1. Introduction and Overview	1
2. Richard McCormick: Ordered Values and Proportionate Reasons	13
McCormick and Neonatal Treatment Decisions	14
McCormick's "Moderate Teleology"	19
Values, Community, and Autonomy: McCormick and Treatment Refusals	28
Goods of Self and Goods of Others: McCormick on Experimentation with Children	31
Proportionate Reason and Consequentialism	35
3. Paul Ramsey: *Agape*, "Covenant Fidelity," and Moral Rules	54
Agape and Covenant Fidelity: Thematic Development	55
Principles, Rules, and 'Exceptions' in Ramsey's Ethics	61
Defective Newborns and "Medical Indications"	65
Medical Indications and Patient Autonomy	74
Covenant-Loyalty in Pediatric Research	81
4. Stanley Hauerwas: Character, Vision, and Narrative in Moral Life	96
The Moral Self in Storied Community	98
Moral Agency, Community, and Medical Treatment Choices for Oneself	110
Suffering, Death, and Caring for Our Children: Hauerwas on Neonatal Treatment Decisions	116
Family, Community, and Medical Experimentation with Children	121
5. James Gustafson: Piety and the Ethics of Theocentric Discernment	130
Theocentrism and Piety	131
Theocentric Ethics: Participation, Discernment, and Relating Parts and Wholes	140
Discernment and the Refusal of Life-Prolonging Treatment	146
Discernment and Treatment Decisions for Defective Neonates	151
Nontherapeutic Pediatric Research: The Good of Parts and of Wholes	155

6. Some Reflections and Suggestions	164
Christian Ethics as Response to Covenant Promise	167
Decisions about Prolonging Our Lives Medically: Reflections on the 'Gift' of Life	172
Neonatal Treatment Decisions: Medical Indications, Parental Autonomy, Distributive Justice, and the Best Interests of Handicapped Infants	180
Children in Nontherapeutic Research: Covenants, Grateful Responses, and the Interests of Children	190
A Postscript	199
Index	203

ACKNOWLEDGEMENTS

This book is a revised form of my doctoral dissertation, entitled "Recent Theological Approaches in Medical Ethics: McCormick, Ramsey, Hauerwas, and Gustafson" (University of Virginia, 1990). Its subject matter was selected in order to reflect two long-standing and dominant areas of interest to me: Christian theology and its ethical manifestations; and moral concerns in the delivery of health care. Theological reflection and discourse have been constant facets of my experience for as long as I can remember; even the 'table-talk' in my parents' home was often focused upon biblical and theological matters. And my interest in health care ethics was sharpened through first-hand encounters and experiences in my employment in several hospital positions during (and between) my college and graduate school years.

The four moralists whose ideas are examined here have all challenged my thinking about theology and medical ethics in profound and varied ways. And each has graciously answered questions that have arisen for me in the research and writing of this book. So, I should begin my thanking Richard McCormick, S.J., Paul Ramsey, Stanley Hauerwas, and James M. Gustafson, whose original ideas and explorations have made this study possible.

I would also like to thank the members of my dissertation committee, Professors Oscar Thorup, David Little, John C. Fletcher, and James F. Childress, for their careful attention and good counsel. I am especially grateful to Professor Childress – teacher and dissertation director extraordinaire – for his generous mentoring, sage advice, and constant friendship and encouragement. He has contributed to this project – and enriched my life – in more ways than I can recount here.

Melody Roberts Aylor, of the University of Virginia, transformed my handwritten and/or poorly typed pages into a computerized and neatly printed dissertation, and I am most grateful for all her hard work. Gloria Albrecht, Gilmary Bauer and Dolores Nieratka, of the University of Detroit Mercy, have read and commented upon parts of this book, and Lisa J. Uchno has proof-read the entire manuscript in its galley form. I am grateful to them and to the University of Detroit Mercy, which allowed me a sabbatical leave in the Fall of 1994 so that I might complete my revisions of this volume. And Earl Shelp, series editor for Kluwer Academic Publishers' *Theology and Medicine* series, has been a constant source of encouragement, advice and good cheer.

Finally, I wish to thank my parents, Lee and Jim Tubbs, to whom this book is dedicated. Their expressions of love, support and concern have enabled the completion of this project in many ways. More importantly, however, their manner of living has shown me much about what an ethic of grace might look like.

CHAPTER ONE

INTRODUCTION AND OVERVIEW

Christian theology has addressed for many centuries the family of issues which we now group under "medical ethics." Care for the sick is encouraged throughout the Hebrew and Christian Scriptures; indeed, Jesus's parable about what it means to be a 'neighbor' – the story of the good Samaritan – is couched in terms of medical care. From the days of the early Church, theologians have developed moral arguments about such issues as contraception, abortion, suicide, euthanasia, and surgical mutilation. And the Church did not comment on such matters from afar: the earliest "hospitals" in the Western world were organized to administer medical (and other) aid as acts of Christian charity. By the early middle ages European hospitals were administered primarily by bishoprics and monasteries, though private lay hospitals appeared by the end of the tenth century [2].

One of the great landmarks in the history of theological ethics – and, by application, medical ethics – is the work of the thirteenth-century philosopher/theologian Thomas Aquinas. Thomas proposed, in his *Summa Theologiae*, a highly systematic natural law theology which has become, in the words of Charles Curran, "the characteristic approach of Roman Catholic moral theology" ([6], p. 1524). Following Thomas, an elaborate scheme of casuistry developed in the Catholic Church in which judgements about moral dilemmas could be deduced from "first principles" of natural law. The continuing vitality of Thomism is clear in such modern pronouncements as Pope Paul VI's much-discussed *Humanae Vitae* (1968), which condemns artificial contraception through a Thomistic deductive methodology and which has helped to stimulate attempts at both reformulation of traditional natural law theology and replacement of it by other, more inductive, personalist, or historically-conscious methodologies. One reformulation of traditional natural law, that proposed by Richard McCormick, will be examined in the next chapter.

Protestant Christianity has done without the elaborate system of Roman Catholic natural law and casuistry, and as a result has produced a wide array of methodologies in theological ethics and a wide range of Protestant "positions" on issues in medical ethics. Reformation emphases on "the freedom of a Christian" and his/her conscience, and the role of the Holy Spirit in illuminating for the believer the will of God through Scripture, have also entailed that the Protestant ethicist has always been guided by "the awareness that he must ever anew invent his casuistry" ([14], p. 1365). Certain theological themes, though, have tended to find dominant positions in modern Protestant ethics – among them *agape* (Christian love-of-neighbor as exemplified in the life and work of Jesus), respect for human life as a *gift* of God, the concept of *stewardship* of God's creation, and *covenant* relation with God (and neighbor). These themes (and others) will be dealt with in later chapters of this volume as we examine the works of Protestant ethicists Paul Ramsey, Stanley Hauerwas, and James Gustafson.

The past 25 years have witnessed an enormous concentration of interest in and discourse about issues in medical ethics – not only (or even primarily) from theological ethicists, but also from moral philosophers, reflective health care professionals, economists, government officials, and a concerned general public. Discussion has produced widely variant perspectives about the very nature of medico-moral dilemmas and methodologies for dealing with them. This volume will explore four recent theological approaches in medical ethics. I have chosen to limit its focus to *theological* approaches because my own interests in ethics grow out of central theological convictions and because I assume the existence of others, with similar commitments, who might benefit from examining with me alternative constructs for applying those commitments to some of the most pressing moral concerns of our time. I use the term "theological *approaches*" because the following explorations will highlight both particular theological-ethical *methods* and also certain theological/anthropological assumptions (or premises) which undergird and shape those methods.[1]

Now, at the outset I must issue something of a disclaimer about the title of this book. For, my topic is not really "Christian theology *and* medical ethics," but, more precisely, "Christian theology *in* medical ethics," or "medical ethics *as* applied theology." This may seem a mere semantic quibble. But I want to avoid from the start the notion that my concern here is with what the 'discipline' of theology might "offer" or "say" to the discipline of medical ethics. In the first place, I think we should steer clear of any suggestion that "medical ethics" is a discrete and autonomous ethical discipline with its own indigenous sets of norms and discursive procedures. Rather, health care as a realm of human activity provides a context, an area of application, for alternative moral visions and claims which are broader than their medical applications. Some moralists have objected to the term "bioethics" for this very reason – namely, that the term seems to suggest a new *kind* of moral reflection rather than simply a locus of application for moral theories, norms, virtues, etc. ([3], p. 9).

Second, even if we clearly define "medical ethics" as an area of concerns within the sub-discipline of applied normative ethics,[2] I think we should still be wary of any language which might imply a chasm between the content and concerns of medical ethics on the one hand and of theology (and theological ethics) on the other. The four theological ethicists whose work will be examined here are not persons who have been trained in two different intellectual disciplines and who want somehow to connect them. They are instead persons whose theological beliefs and perspectives have shaped their conceptions and models of moral life, and who have explicated their theological moralities through discussions of particular issues and problems faced in the field of medical care and research. So my title is actually an abbreviation for a more accurate but utterly unwieldly one: "Recent Theological Conceptions of Moral Life and Judgement, Particularly as Developed in the Context of Decision-Making in Biomedicine".[3]

The four moralists dealt with in this study were selected for several reasons. First, they are all quite simply "leading" figures in the literature of biomedical ethics. They have participated in ongoing published discussions of key medico-moral issues, and have been invited to contribute their analyses for public policy-making deliberations as well. Second, for practical purposes, the extent of their various publications makes available to us a large sampling of works which illustrate both substantive and methodological positions taken by each of them. And third, their particular approaches provide analytically interesting contrasts, in that they emphasize different aspects of moral life (e.g., morality of values, intrinsic morality of actions, and perspectives and qualities of moral agents themselves).

Richard A. McCormick, S.J., is John A. O'Brien Professor of Christian Ethics at Notre Dame University. From 1965 until 1984 he wrote the influential "Notes on Moral Theology" series in *Theological Studies* (and he still contributes to that series). McCormick is a leading figure among Roman Catholic moral theologians who have suggested that a teleological model of moral life and natural law are indeed implicit within the Aristotelian-Thomistic Catholic moral tradition. His view is that actions are to be judged as to how they promote or attack values within the objective hierarchy of values (*ordo bonorum*): there should exist a proper "proportion" between value sacrificed and value realized in any moral choice.

Paul Ramsey, former Harrington Spear Paine Professor of Christian Ethics at Princeton University, was, before his death in 1988, perhaps the most prolific contemporary Christian ethicist in terms of contributions to the literature of theology and medical ethics. Ramsey's first and most systematic treatment of theological ethics was his *Basic Christian Ethics* (1950). Since then he has addressed insightfully such diverse issues as civil disobedience, just war, genetic intervention and experimentation, research involving human subjects, abortion, and care for the dying. Central to Ramsey's work is the notion of "covenant fidelity" between persons, derived in his view from the biblical concept of *agape* and modelled upon God's own covenant-righteousness. Obedience to (and imitation of) God takes a consistently deontological form in Ramsey's thought: obligation to fulfill the unconditional, rule-expressed norms of covenant fidelity, rather than a weighing of "goods" or "values" to be realized in concrete situations of choice, is, for him, the form of Christian ethics.

Stanley Hauerwas, Professor of Theological Ethics at the Divinity School, Duke University, is at the vanguard of a movement in theological ethics which describes Christian moral life in terms of the "character" and "virtues" of moral agents (and communities). The central ethical question in this view is not, "What should we do?" but rather, "Who should we be?" Hauerwas argues that an exclusive emphasis on ethical dilemmas and decision-making, whether within a value-dominant or a rule-dominant method, isolates a particular aspect of moral life as the *whole* of morality, when in reality we should be attentive to a broader and richer moral project: the formation and expression of moral character. As we will see, Hauerwas employs the aesthetic notions of "vision" and "narrative" in explaining the acquisition of virtue and development of moral character.

James M. Gustafson, Henry R. Luce Professor of Humanities and Comparative Studies at Emory University, is highly respected not only for his own particular approach in moral reflection but also for his clear and insightful analyses and critiques of Protestantism's "simplistic Christian moralisms." For many years he has sought to stress, in his own words, "the importance of taking very seriously the kinds of precise and technical information required to make particular judgments and choices (while not losing sight of the difficulties in getting accurate information and ideologically unbiased interpretation), and the importance of making the moral arguments of Christians more rigorous both philosophically and theologically" [12]. Indeed, readers of Gustafson's essays concerning particular moral dilemmas (such as abortion or the non-feeding of defective newborns) must surely be impressed by the thoroughness with which the author probes all relevant information and options before suggesting any conclusions. Recently Gustafson has produced a systematic expression of his own theological-ethical approach – the two-volume *Ethics From a Theocentric Perspective* (1981, 1984). In that work he refines and clarifies a view which emphasizes the primacy of *piety* in Christian life – piety which rescues ethics from anthropocentrism and enables us to "discern" the divine will and "participate" in the divine ordering of creation such that we "relate ourselves and all things in a manner appropriate to their relations to God."

These four moralists, then, represent a range of substantive assumptions and reflective methodologies for our consideration. Their views will be addressed individually in each of the next four chapters.

Now, in any comparative study dealing with subject-matter so broad as to encompass theological beliefs and ethical methodologies, some particular 'benchmarks' or 'reference-points' are needed as a way into each of the approaches. For this study, I have chosen three much-debated issues in medical ethics to serve as 'moral prisms' and to provide a structural backbone for chapters 2–5: (1) treatment decisions about 'defective' (i.e., severely malformed or genetically diseased) infants; (2) refusals of life-prolonging medical treatment by competent adults; and (3) the use of children in medical experimentation which is 'non-therapeutic' (i.e., which promises no direct medical benefit for the individual subject-child). These issues have been discussed in the literature, more or less fully, by each of our compared thinkers. Further, and more importantly, these particular issues are highly *representative*, in that the kinds of concerns they force us to take into account are also applicable to many other dilemmas within (and outside of) the health care context.

Medical treatment of defective newborns has become a matter of intense moral – and political – debate in the public forum. Numerous physicians, philosophers and theologians have contributed to the debate stirred by the now-famous "Johns Hopkins case" in the early 1970's. In that instance, the parents of a newborn infant with Down's syndrome and duodenal atresia (blockage of the small intestine) refused permission for surgical correction of their child's intestinal problem. As a result, the infant died of starvation/dehydration after 15 days of life because his duodenal atresia made feeding impossible. The parents felt that the special problems of a Down's child (especially mental retardation) would have rendered their son's life a disvalue to him and a burden to the rest of the family. A 1973 article in the *New England Journal of Medicine* by physicians Raymond Duff and A.G.M. Campbell of the Yale-New Haven Medical Center dispelled any notion that the Johns Hopkins case represented an isolated instance of parental/professional choice against treatment of infants. Duff and Campbell described how, of 299 infant deaths in their Neonatal Intensive Care Unit over a 17-month period, 43 deaths followed a deliberate choice by parents and/or physicians to withhold or withdraw life-prolonging medical treatment because continued life was not seen to be in the infant's best interests [8].

Perhaps the best-known catalyst of public debate about neonatal treatment decisions was the Bloomington, Indiana "Baby Doe case" (1982). As in the Johns Hopkins case, the parents of Down's-afflicted Baby Doe refused consent for surgery to correct a condition (tracheo-esophageal fistula) which prevented feeding him. He died after 6 days of non-feeding. Reagan administration officials interpreted Baby Doe's non-treatment as discrimination against a handicapped person, and announced policies to restrict similar choices. Several of these "Baby Doe Rules" were subsequently overturned by the courts, and finally the U.S. Supreme Court in 1986, as unjustifiable federal intrusions into parental and medical decision-making.

But both houses of the U.S. Congress also proferred bills concerning selective nontreatment of handicapped infants. Compromise legislation, known as the Child Abuse Amendments of 1984, passed in September, 1984. That law amended the Child Abuse Prevention and Treatment Act of 1974 (Public Law 98–457) by redefining child abuse and neglect to include the "withholding of medically indicated treatment from handicapped infants with life-threatening conditions" [9]. "Medically indicated treatment" was defined as whatever the treating physicians deem "most likely to be effective in ameliorating or correcting" the infant's life-threatening conditions. Treatment (other than "appropriate nutrition, hydration, and medication") is *not* considered medically indicated only when: (a) the infant is "chronically and irreversibly comatose"; (b) the provision of such treatment "would merely prolong dying, not be effective in ameliorating or correcting all of the infant's life-threatening conditions, or otherwise be futile in terms of the survival of the infant"; or (c) the provision of such treatment "would be virtually futile in terms of the survival of the infant and the treatment itself under such circumstances would be inhumane."

These guidelines were aimed primarily at state governments, to be applied in enforcing their individual child abuse and neglect statutes. The only direct penalty attached is the withdrawal of federal child abuse program monies for states whose hospitals are found to be allowing treatment choices on grounds other than those defined above. Even so, the 1984 legislation has come under much criticism. The American Medical Association, for example, holds that the legislation does not consider fully the "quality of life" of severely handicapped infants who *do* survive with aggressive treatment [1].

Moreover, various state court rulings handed down since 1984 would appear to allow somewhat more leeway in neonatal treatment decisions than the federal legislation prescribes. In my state (Michigan), for instance, judicial precedent for such decisions was established by the Michigan Court of Appeals in its 1992 *Rosebush* ruling [17]. The court held that for all incompetent patients with no medical probability of "substantial recovery" and whose treatment preferences cannot be known, decisions for or against life-prolonging treatment should be based on the patient's "best interests." Specifically, the court stated (citing the New Jersey Supreme Court's *Conroy* decision) that a determination of the patient's best interests should take into account: evidence about his/her "present level of physical, sensory, emotional and cognitive functioning"; the degree of physical pain resulting from treatment (or non-treatment); the degree of "humiliation, dependence, and loss of dignity" probably resulting from the patient's condition or from treatment options; life expectancy and prognosis for recovery with or without treatment; and the general benefits, risks and side effects of treatment options under consideration.

Of course, legislative and judicial prescriptions for decisions to treat defective newborns are not our central concern here; our focus is upon theological-ethical reasoning about such decisions. But the points of view described in the previous paragraphs are, as we will see, substantively similar to some of the normative positions examined in the next four chapters. Argumentative positions advanced in the public forum on this issue are often oversimplified and sloganized: some are said to be advocating a "sanctity of life" position; others a position sensitive to "quality of life" or "meaningful life" considerations; and still others a notion (drawn from legal parlance) of "due care" for all those in need of medical assistance. Each of these general positions is represented to some extent in the following chapters. Behind the slogans, though, lie basic theological concerns and questions. We might ask, for instance, What is the proper interpretation of human life and death? For if we have theological reasons to dread physical death and/or to exult in physical life for its own sake, then our general attitude toward prolonging (suffering) life – our own and others' – will be different than if we interpret life in the world as, say, merely a "vale of tears." Further, we might ask, Under what conditions, if any, might we say that what makes human life 'human' is no longer present? (Or, in terminology which will become more familiar shortly, When can we say that human life has "fulfilled its potential?") Finally, if we acknowledge a divinely-mandated duty to love those around us, how do we interpret the loving "care" we owe to those in need of aid? Should we define "care" in terms of what *results* our actions can produce for the other person, or perhaps in terms of what our caring-actions *symbolize* or *express* toward the other?

In sum, then, the issue of treatment for defective newborns will be our way into central theological-ethical concerns about the meaning of 'human' physical life and about the nature and limits of 'caring' for it.

The second prismatic issue dealt with comparatively here will be that of refusals of life-prolonging medical treatment (by competent persons). Such refusals are often painfully controversial in our society because they bring into conflict cherished social values. On the one hand, our collective view of social structures (and the role of government) has strongly liberal roots; we honor individual freedoms highly. The value of autonomous freedom relating to treatment of one's body was cited by the Supreme Court of Kansas in its 1960 ruling in *Natanson* v. *Kline*: Justice Alfred Schroeder wrote, for the majority, that

Anglo-American law starts with the premise of thorough-going self-determination. It follows that each man is considered to be master of his own body, and he may, if he be of sound mind, expressly prohibit the performance of life-saving surgery, or other medical treatment [15].

Thirty years later, a federal constitutional basis for Justice Schroeder's argument was affirmed by the U.S. Supreme Court in its now-famous *Cruzan* decision (1990). Chief Justice William Rehnquist, writing for the majority, noted that a constitutionally-protected "liberty-interest" in refusing unwanted medical treatment may be inferred from the Fourteenth Amendment (and from prior court decisions) [4]. Just a few months after the *Cruzan* ruling Congress passed the "Patient Self-Determination Act," requiring health care institutions to inform their clients (and the community) about their right to elect/reject life-prolonging medical treatment via advance directives [16].

On the other hand, though, we often sense something unbearably tragic, perhaps even perverse, in some choices against preserving one's life.[4] So the moral question becomes, When is the freedom (or 'right') of self-determination in health care 'rightly' to be exercised; or when may it rightly be limited? (In practice, of course, it is most often limited by means of withholding information from a patient about her/his treatment options. Despite legislative and judicial emphases on the "right to refuse treatment," a recent large survey of health professionals caring for the terminally ill found that informed involvement of patients in decisions regarding their treatment is more the exception than the norm. Of 1446 professionals responding, only 31% agreed with the statement that "Staff find out what critically and terminally ill patients want"; 33% felt that patients understand information they are given about their condition/treatment options; and 33% felt that patients "get the help they need to make decisions about care alternatives." Interestingly, 47% admitted to acting "against my conscience" in providing care for the terminally ill, and 55% regarded the treatment they have provided some patients as "overly burdensome" [18].

The medical community – historic battlers for cures and/or palliative means for *life's* improvement and extension – have, understandably, often tended to view refusals of life-prolonging treatment as irrational and wrong. And conflicts between patients' desires to refuse life-saving therapy and health professionals' desires to provide it are sometimes seen as pitting a "right to die" against a "duty to treat."

In the early 1980's, the case of Elizabeth Bouvia provided a good example of this conflict. Mrs. Bouvia, a 26 year old cerebral palsy victim with nearly complete paralysis and painful arthritis, considered her life not worth living and chose to end it by the only available means not requiring direct assistance from others – starvation. She asked to be allowed to remain in her local hospital and receive hygienic care and pain medication but no other food or medicine. The hospital refused, and Mrs. Bouvia brought suit. The original court ruling stated that "she does have a fundamental right to terminate her own life, but this right has been overcome by the strong interest of the state and society . . . Our society values life" [5]. In subsequently permitting the hospital to force-feed Mrs. Bouvia, Judge John H. Hews explained that he had also considered the interests of third parties: the health care professionals "who would have to assist in her demise" if she were allowed a fatal fast; other disabled persons "similarly situated" (for whom a poor precedent would presumably be set); and the medical profession itself, whose "integrity" the state has an interest in maintaining [13].

While the court was concerned to adjudicate between conflicting legal rights and interests, Mrs. Bouvia's lawyer described her situation in somewhat different terms by claiming that she does not "have the obligation to endure what to her is unendurable" [13]. The existence and stringency of such an obligation – and its possible foundations – will be the focus of discussions of treatment refusal in the next four chapters. In theological terms, this issue invokes powerfully notions of human *freedom* within the created order and human *responsibility* to God (and, derivatively, to other persons). As in the issue of treatment for defective newborns, claims about "respect for life" and "quality of life" enter into refusal-of-treatment discussions. But in the latter case we must also struggle with the question of how much autonomous freedom should be respected/limited in persons who have made "quality of life" decisions about their own lives. Can the choice to hasten the end of one's life be entailed by "the freedom of a Christian?"

All four of the theological ethicists examined here hold that persons can rightly – and should be allowed to – choose to reject life-prolonging medical therapy in some circumstances. We will also see, though, that all four reject the notion that every rational person properly has (or should be allowed) an unlimited freedom to choose against life whenever life becomes too personally burdensome.

The third medico-moral issue to be highlighted in this study – children's participation in nontherapeutic research – involves not life-or-death decisions but rather allocation decisions for the 'costs' of medical progress. Should we allow the involvement of children in research which promises them no medical benefit but which will generate knowledge useful in treating other, larger populations of children? As most commentators point out (e.g., [11]), this issue is more complex than the general issue of adult participation in research for several reasons. First, young children are not simply 'little adults' physiologically. Their metabolic and drug-response pathways, for example, are so un-adult that quite often the results of experimentation with adult subjects are not safely applicable in pediatric treatment. Thus, experimentation with children can be the only way to remove the guesswork from treating children. Second, and similarly, some diseases strike only children; so it would be impossible to study treatment modalities for these diseases in adults. But, third, the hazards or harms of experimentation may also be greater for young subjects than for adults. A routine venipuncture, for example, is a minor inconvenience for (most) adults but could be quite traumatic for a child. And fourth, a fully voluntary, informed consent to participation in research is generally unavailable from a child.

These factors have been afforded varying weights in public policy decisions concerning nontherapeutic research in children. The Medical Research Council of Great Britain, for instance, has declared that, "parents and guardians of minors cannot give consent on their behalf to any procedures which are of no particular benefit to them and which may carry some risk of harm" [7]. On the other hand, the U.S. Department of Health and Human Services has issued regulations, applicable to "all research involving children as subjects, conducted or supported by" the D.H.H.S., which allow relatively more leeway for approval of research by the Institutional Review Boards (IRBs) of individual research facilities [10]. Local IRBs may approve nontherapeutic research which does not involve "greater than minimal risk" to the children-subjects if adequate provisions have been made for soliciting the child's assent[5] and the parents' or guardian's consent (and if other substantive standards for subject-safety and withdrawal privileges are met). Further, research "not otherwise approvable" which presents "a reasonable opportunity to further the understanding, prevention, or alleviation of a serious problem affecting the health or welfare of children" may also be allowed if it meets assent/consent criteria, will be conducted "in accordance with sound ethical principles," and is approved not only by the local IRB but also by the Secretary of D.H.H.S, "after consultation with a panel of experts in pertinent disciplines . . . and following opportunity for public review and comment" ([10], p. 9819). In short, the D.H.H.S. regulations, in contrast to their British counterpart, are more fully *procedural*: proxy consent is acceptable, and allowable weights of possible risks and benefits are determined on a case-by-case basis at several regulatory levels in the D.H.H.S.

Nontherapeutic research involving children raises at least two interrelated moral questions, one having to do with the research itself and the other with the role of the subject. First, to what extent is it justifiable to place a small group of subjects at risk in order to benefit another (larger) group of persons? Does 'respect' for individual persons entail an absolute refusal to incur *any* risk of harm to particular subjects in any possible nontherapeutic trial? Or, does it perhaps entail a concern for present and future sick persons which would allow at least small risks to some other subject-persons on their behalf?[6]

This leads to the second question: If nontherapeutic research can be justified because of its potential benefits, then what is the nature of any given individual's obligation (if any) to be a research subject and thus to benefit other persons? This is, obviously, a central concern in situations where the potential subject is incompetent to consent (because of age or mental infirmity) and we cannot know with certainty whether he/she would choose to volunteer if competent to do so, and for what reasons. For, if we consider the acceptance of (small) personal risks in order to help others to be a duty we all share, then we might have a reasonable basis for assuming that incompetent potential subjects would volunteer if they could. But no such assumption is possible if we consider the bearing of *any* risk for the sake of another to be an act of supererogatory beneficence; and we would be hard-pressed to justify any recruitment of incompetents from this perspective.

These moral questions about children in research have deeply theological roots. What, we might ask, is the proper relation between the good of individual persons and the good of the human community (or the good of all God's creation)? What does it mean to participate responsibly in the created order? Is participation in nontherapeutic research to be seen as an act of charity; and, if so, is it something we should expect or require of all persons? We will see in the following chapters that these questions have found varied answers among Christian ethicists; thus their normative policy positions differ as well. Three of our four selected thinkers (Ramsey, McCormick and Hauerwas) have engaged in lengthy published debate about children's participation in nontherapeutic research, and their arguments reveal theological premises as diverse as their substantive conclusions.

These three issues, then – treatment of defective newborns, autonomous refusals of treatment, and children in nontherapeutic research – will provide common reference-points for examining the theological ethics of McCormick, Ramsey, Hauerwas and Gustafson. Each of these prismatic issues will help illuminate not only differing theological 'starting points' (presumptions and premises about God, human beings, and the created 'world') but also differing methods of arriving at moral judgements. My purpose in what follows is critical as well as comparative. So, inasmuch as the moral methodologies considered here can be seen to be representative of particular 'theories' of morality such as 'teleology,' 'deontology' and 'virtue-ethics,' I will refer at various points to relevant criticisms of those theoretical formulations by moral philosophers and theologians.

This book's final chapter will be largely reflective. In it I will pull together some criticisms and conclusions from chapters 2–5 in order to formulate my own reflective response to the three prismatic issues described above. I make no claim, of course, to offer the 'final word' of Christian ethics on these subjects. This volume is an exploration – a critical exploration by one Christian ethicist of the impressive work of four others. So, its larger purpose is to clarify and compare ethical 'options' in and for a community of theologically concerned persons.

NOTES

[1] I am assuming, for analytical purposes, a simple distinction between "theology" as the reflective task of demonstrating the realities of God, human persons, and the 'world' (and their interrelationships), and "theological ethics" as the reflective task of moving from these realities to a discernment (through a "method" as I am using the term) of what is morally 'good,' 'right,' 'virtuous,' 'obligatory,' etc.

[2] As distinguished from 'descriptive ethics' or 'metaethics.'

[3] "Biomedicine" is a term which has been coined to indicate the professional areas of both health care delivery per se and biological-medical research involving human subjects (undertaken to produce knowledge which will improve health care). Thus, the term "medical ethics" is often taken to have a restricted referent (i.e., restricted to moral issues in medical treatment and practice) when compared to the broader term "biomedical ethics." But I will use the simpler, more familiar "medical ethics" in this volume to refer to moral reflection on praxis in both health care delivery and biomedical experimentation.

[4] Of course, not every choice against life-preserving treatment can be said to be a choice against continued life. For example, the Jehovah's Witness patient who refuses blood transfusions desires not to die but simply to avoid sinning against God by 'consuming' the forbidden blood. Also,

when can we say that a refusal of life-prolonging treatment merits the highly evaluative designation of 'suicide'? Definitions of suicide vary, and discussions of treatment-refusals are often lumped together with discussions of the morality of suicide without clear conceptual distinctions being made. Some suggested conceptual linkages between suicide and refusal of life-prolonging treatment will be examined for each of the theological-ethical approaches dealt with in the next four chapters.

⁵ But, if the IRB "determines that the capability of some or all the children is so limited that they cannot reasonably be consulted . . . the assent of the children is not a necessary condition for proceeding with the research" ([10], p. 9819).

⁶ Maurice Visscher has argued that the moral "first function" of physicians is to "do no harm," and that only medical experimentation can make this possible, since physicians must first *find out* what will or will not probably be harmful (or helpful) to patients before they can truly refrain from harm in clinical interventions. (See [19], esp. Chapter 3)

REFERENCES

1. 'Accord Reached on Rules for Care in "Baby Doe" Case': July 4, 1984, *New York Times*, pp. A1+.
2. Amundson, D.W.: 1978, 'Medical Ethics, History of: Medieval Europe: Fourth to Sixteenth Century', in W. Reich (ed.), *Encyclopedia of Bioethics*, vol. 3, The Free Press, New York, pp. 938–50.
3. Beauchamp, T.L. and Childress, J.F.: 1983, *Principles of Biomedical Ethics*, 2nd ed., Oxford University Press, New York.
4. *Cruzan v. Director of Missouri Department of Health*: 26 June, 1990, U.S. Supreme Court, 58 LW 4916.
5. Cummings, J.: Dec. 17, 1983, 'Plea by Patient for Starvation Barred by Court', *New York Times*, p. A8.
6. Curran, C.E.: 1978, 'Roman Catholicism', in W. Reich (ed.), *Encyclopedia of Bioethics*, vol. 4, The Free Press, New York, pp. 1522–33.
7. Curran, W.J. and Beecher, H.: 1969, 'Experimentation in Children', *Journal of the American Medical Association* 210, 77–83.
8. Duff, R. and Campbell, A.G.M.: 1973, 'Moral and Ethical Dilemmas in the Special Care Nursery', *New England Journal of Medicine* 289, 890–94.
9. *Federal Register*: April 15, 1985, 14878–14892.
10. *Federal Register*: March 8, 1983 (48 FR 9814).
11. Fost, N.C.: 1978, 'Children and Biomedicine', in W. Reich (ed.), *Encyclopedia of Bioethics*, vol. 1, The Free Press, New York, pp. 150–56.
12. Gustafson, J.M.: 1980, 'A Theocentric Interpretation of Life', *The Christian Century* 97, 754–60.
13. Hughes, W.G. and Belcher, J.: Dec. 16, 1983, 'Right to Starve Plea Denied', *Los Angeles Times*, p. I-1.
14. Johnson, J.T.: 1978, 'Protestantism: History of Protestant Medical Ethics', in W. Reich (ed.), *Encyclopedia of Bioethics*, vol. 3, The Free Press, New York, pp. 1364–72.
15. *Natanson v. Kline*: 1960, 186 Kan. 393, 350 P. 2d. 1093.
16. Omnibus Budget Reconciliation Act of 1990, Title IV, Sec. 4206: Oct. 26, 1990, *Congressional Record*, 12638.
17. *Rosebush v. Oakland County Prosecutor*: 1992, 195 Mich. App. 675, 491 N.W.2d. 633.
18. Solomon, M.Z. et al.: 1993, 'Decisions Near the End of Life: Professional Views on Life-Sustaining Treatments', *American Journal of Public Health* 83/1, 14–23.
19. Visscher, M.: 1975, *Ethical Constraints and Imperatives in Medical Research*, Charles C. Thomas, Springfield, IL.

CHAPTER TWO

RICHARD McCORMICK: ORDERED VALUES AND PROPORTIONATE REASONS

The backbone of Roman Catholic moral theology is the concept of 'natural law' (*lex naturae*) – objective moral claims known (to some extent, at least) to all persons by their very nature as human beings, application of which may be derived through discursive reasoning.[1] Timothy O'Connell has described, in a simplified but useful way, two different sources of the notion of natural law in intellectual history ([52], Chapter 13). One of these sources, which he refers to as the "Greek" source, conceived of natural law as "precisely the objective demand placed on humankind to conform to the givenness of reality." In this view, the cosmos was seen to be rigid, static, and unyielding, with human survival depending upon "cooperation with the rhythms of life." So, in other words, the dictates of reason were seen to be "out there" in nature, to be observed and followed. The other conceptual source of natural law – the "Roman" source – tended to place reason fully in the human self. O'Connell cites Cicero, for example, as emphasizing the "natural" as "right reason, human intelligence, prudent and thoughtful action directed to humane ends." This is no "abject capitulation to the facts of life," but rather a willingness to use intelligence and common sense to solve life's riddles and control life's caprices.

Thomas Aquinas (and the Thomistic tradition of moral theology which followed him) seem to have vacillated between the 'order of nature' and 'order of reason' conceptions of natural law. O'Connell cites Thomas's assertion that, "to the natural law belongs those things to which a man is inclined naturally: and among these it is proper to man to be inclined to act according to reason" (from the *Summa Theologiae* I–II, 94, 4). But Thomas also included under the rubric of natural law the demand to conform to animal facticity, and referred to natural law as "common to all animals" (*ST* I–II, 95,4). Thomas's systematic theology was teleological in character, stressing the natural and eternal "ends" of human beings; and man's rational orientation of self in accordance with those ends was a central theme of it. (He considered "prudence" to be the crowning virtue of the rational soul.) But in dealing with certain concrete ethical issues – especially issues of sexuality and procreation – Thomas tended to identify natural law with biological and physical processes.[2]

Within the past few decades there has been intense interest among Catholic moral theologians in re-examining and reformulating Thomistic natural law in terms of both its formal principles and its metaphysical foundations. Some of these theologians have re-emphasized what O'Connell calls the "Greek" influence in Thomism – which would, for instance, prohibit some actions as "intrinsically evil" inasmuch as they are seen to corrupt a 'natural' function or relationship.[3] Others have emphasized the historical nature of human experience and understanding, and have stressed the contextual and consequence-recognizing side of Thomistic rationality (the "Roman" influence). Richard McCormick, the subject of this chapter, fits more fully into the latter group. He suggests that a 'proportional' approach to weighing the values we seek to affirm in our moral choices has been implicit all along in the Aristotelian-Thomistic teleology of intelligible ends of human pursuit. And his model of moral decision-making includes justification of exceptions to abstract moral norms according to particular concrete circumstances (or, more precisely, when there exists a positive proportion between a value to be realized and a value sacrificed by a particular choice). The specifics of his moral methodology will be examined in Section 2, below, after we begin with a brief account of his views on one very compelling sort of value-conflict: the concrete issue of selective nontreatment of defective newborns.

1. McCORMICK AND NEONATAL TREATMENT DECISIONS

Traditional Catholic moral theology has maintained for many centuries that the obligation to prolong human physical life is not an absolute obligation; there are limits to the duty of continued living.[4] Long before the question of whether life should be sustained indefinitely via medical technology was even considered, the Catholic Church had formulated criteria for distinguishing between life-sustaining means which could be deemed 'ordinary' and those deemed 'extraordinary.' In terms of theological-moral judgements about decisions for or against treatment, a great deal of weight rested upon this distinction. For, to choose against an 'ordinary' means of preserving one's life was to choose for suicide (a mortal sin), while a choice against 'extraordinary' means was considered a responsible exercise of human freedom. Likewise, to choose against the former on behalf of an incompetent patient (whose own wishes cannot be known) would be tantamount to murder; to choose against the latter would merely be allowing that person to die without further annoyance, and could be morally justifiable.

The tradition has generally held that 'ordinary' means are those medicines, treatments, or interventions which can be obtained and used without excessive hardship to the patient and which offer a reasonable hope of benefitting the patient; 'extraordinary' means are those whose use would cause excessive hardship to the patient and/or would offer little hope of benefit. So, two criteria are included in the ordinary/extraordinary means distinction: a prospect-of-benefit criterion and a criterion of 'hardship' relative to expected benefit. The reasoning behind the prospect-of-benefit factor is obvious: one is not morally required to undergo therapy which is clearly an exercise in futility. To require such therapy would be purely vitalistic, and the tradition has never held that biological 'life' is humankind's final end. The 'hardship' factor historically has been open to quite an array of considerations. In the days before antisepsis and anesthesia, for example, major surgery (such as amputation) would certainly count as a grave hardship for the physical agony it entailed (as well as its bleak prospect-of-benefit). Exorbitant financial cost of life-preserving care was another consideration sometimes cited in determining that continued treatment was morally optional ('extraordinary'). Gerald Kelly has pointed out that classical moral theologians also included under "grave hardship" fundamental inconveniences to one's established lifestyle; for example, moving to another climate or country in order to preserve one's life was considered more than God would demand of people "whose lives were, so to speak, rooted in the land, and whose native town or village was as dear as life itself, and for whom, moreover, travel was always difficult and often dangerous" ([28], p. 132).

With the rise of modern medical technology, the traditional ordinary/extraordinary means distinction has become much more complicated. Originally, the criterion of prospect-of-benefit meant prospect of success in curing or remedying the patient's medical problem, thus sustaining life. But now that we can mechanically preserve cardio-pulmonary 'life' almost indefinitely for so many patients, is it really a 'benefit' to them to do so? And what counts as excessive hardship when so many treatment modalities are readily available? Despite new conceptual difficulties with the traditional distinction, the language of ordinary and extraordinary means still holds a position of wide acceptance in medical ethics. The American Medical Association, for example, employed that language in its 1973 position statement on mercy-killing (which the A.M.A. condemned) and letting die: "The cessation of the employment of extraordinary means to prolong the life of the body when there is irrefutable evidence that biological death is imminent is the decision of the patient and/or his immediate family. The advice and judgement of the physician should be freely available to the patient and/or his immediate family."[5]

Richard McCormick is one of many medical ethicists who have suggested that the language of "ordinary and extraordinary means" has outlived its usefulness – that it leads too many to focus too quickly on whether or not a treatment is medically 'usual.' McCormick favors instead the terms "reasonable and unreasonable treatment," and, as we will see, favors a substantive standard of reasonableness involving 'quality of life' considerations in decision-making about treatment of the incompetent ill (including defective newborns).

The most appropriate starting point for gaining an understanding of McCormick's position on this issue is his view of the theological significance of human biological life and death. The Judeo-Christian tradition has, in his opinion, consistently sought to steer a course between medical vitalism and medical pessimism (which would entail a willingness to kill "when life seems frustrating, burdensome, 'useless'") – both of which represent an "idolatry of life." Behind this "middle course" is an attitude that "life is indeed a basic and precious good, but a good to be preserved precisely as the condition of other values" ([38], p. 345). McCormick frequently cites with approval Pope Pius XII's statement that, "[l]ife, death, all temporal activities are in fact subordinated to spiritual ends."[6] And what are these spiritual ends? First, there may be particular "higher goods" for which one might legitimately sacrifice one's life, such as "glory of God, salvation of souls, service of one's brethren, etc." ([40], p. 321). But, second, the overall "meaning, substance, and consummation of life from the Judeo-Christian perspective" is the love of God and love of neighbor (for the latter love is "in some very real sense" our love of God). God demands to be recognized and loved by us in others. From this it follows, for McCormick, that life's meaning, substance, and consummation are to be found in human *relationships* (and the "qualities of justice, respect, concern, compassion, and support that surround them") ([38], p. 346). Other values, for which life is the conditional value, are rooted in or cluster around human relationships; thus the capacity or potential for human relationships is a minimal condition for truly 'human' life. Where the capacity or potential for human relationships is absent, "that life can be said to have achieved its potential" ([38], p. 349).

This understanding of the primacy of "relational potential" is at the center of McCormick's reformulation of the ordinary vs. extraordinary means distinction. In his reflections on treatment of defective newborns he describes two applications of his relational potential criterion which roughly parallel the traditional prospect-of-benefit and hardship/benefit criteria. First, treatment is unreasonable and thus morally optional when the patient has no potential for human relationships at all (as in the case of an anencephalic infant or one who will never be conscious). Second, treatment might also be unreasonable and not morally required for persons whose potential for human relationships "would be so threatened, strained, or submerged that they would no longer function as the heart and meaning of the individual's life as they should" (or, in other words, "would be utterly submerged and undeveloped in the mere struggle to survive") ([38], p. 349; [53], p. 316). A badly malformed infant in constant pain, for example, might be unable to relate to others because of the intensity of his/her suffering.

McCormick is clear that these applications of a relational potential criterion – particularly the latter application – involve 'quality of life' judgements; but he is also certain that failure to consider what *kind* of 'life' we are preserving technologically is a form of medical vitalism "that makes no human or Judeo-Christian sense." The hidden danger in quality of life judgements is that they may become differential 'quality of *persons*' judgements. McCormick is careful to point out that every person is of equal value; but 'life' as a metabolic condition may not be equally 'valuable' to persons in terms of its relational possibilities (or lack thereof). Further, he reminds us that life's potentiality for other values (through relationships) is dependent upon both "external factors" (such as one's socio-economic status, one's family situation, etc.) and "the very condition of the individual." Negative external factors "we can and must change. That is what social justice is all about." It is only the physical *condition* of the individual – and the relational potential it allows – which is the proper focus and limit of 'quality of life' judgements.

Some practical ramifications of this notion of quality of life evaluations based upon relational potential are outlined in a 1983 article co-authored by McCormick and John Paris, S.J. [53], in which the following guidelines are offered for treatment/nontreatment of defective infants: (1) Managerial or institutional reasons (including the family's ability to cope with a disabled baby) are not sufficient for omitting life-saving interventions. It is "an unacceptable erosion of our respect for life to make the gift of life once given depend on the personalities and emotional or financial capacities of the parents alone." (2) Retardation alone does not justify withholding life-sustaining treatment. (3) Life-preserving intervention may be omitted or withdrawn "when there is excessive hardship on the patient, especially when this combines with poor prognosis (e.g., repeated cardiac surgery, low prognosis transplants, increasingly iatrogenic oxygenation for low birthweight babies)." (4) Such interventions also may be omitted or withdrawn "at a point when it becomes clear that expected life can be had only for a relatively brief time and only with the continued use of artificial feeding (e.g., some cases of necrotizing enterocolitis)" ([53], p. 316; see also [41], pp. 144–49). As the last two of these guidelines illustrate, McCormick's notion of *when* relational potential would be "utterly submerged and undeveloped in the mere struggle to survive" correlates closely with the traditional conception of 'grave hardship' (relative to expected benefit) by which a given medical treatment may be judged 'extraordinary.' However, it is also clear that his evaluative standard of relational potential might apply in cases where none of the traditional conceptions of 'grave hardship' apply – as, presumably, in the case of a severely deformed and mentally retarded child who is *not* in great pain or requiring endless painful treatments but nevertheless fits the prognostic criterion of no prospect for relational potential.[7]

Taking into account McCormick's view of human biological life as a "relative good" and his insistence that we must make quality of life judgements based on some conception of what makes human life genuinely 'human,' a critic might well ask whether he is not perhaps building a case against what we know as the principle of the 'sanctity of human life.' However, McCormick insists that his approach cannot be viewed in this manner:

Actually, the two approaches ought not to be set against each other . . . Quality of life assessments ought to made within an over-all reverence for life, as an extension of one's respect for the sanctity of life. However, there are times when preserving the life of one with no capacity for those aspects of life that we regard as *human* is a violation of the sanctity of life itself. Thus to separate the two approaches and call one *sanctity* of life, the other *quality* of life, is a false conceptual split that very easily suggests that the term 'sanctity of life' is being used in an exhortatory way ([38], p. 397).

Further, he also insists that viewing human life as a "relative good" does not reduce it to a *bonum utile* (a "useful" and "negotiable" good). Rather, he speaks of our duties toward preserving a *bonum honestum* (life as a "good in itself"), recognizing that these duties "may differ depending upon the conditions of that *bonum honestum*" ([38], p. 395).

The process of decision-making for or against treatment of defective infants must focus, in McCormick's view, on "the child's good, this alone." He is aware of the caveat that it is "all but impossible for *healthy adults* to extrapolate backward on what kind of life will be acceptable to the infant." Nevertheless, "if we are to avoid vitalism in practice, these judgements must sometimes be made" ([38], p. 400). Procedurally, such judgements are the "onerous prerogative" of those persons who bear responsibility for the welfare of the family – the parents (in consultation with physicians). And McCormick allows that, given the difficulty of making a "reasonable" assessment of what the child would want, "a certain range of choice must be allowed to parents, a certain margin of error, a certain space" ([53], p. 316; [41], p. 148). Even so, the parents' moral judgement of what is reasonable in their child's case should also seem clear and reasonable to the rest of us as well (for, "ethical persons ought to be reason-giving persons"). When parents choose a course that is "questionably no longer in the best interests of the infant," then society has a duty to intervene ([53], p. 316). McCormick and Paris suggest that the best societal oversight for parents' decisions would be a broadly-based interdisciplinary hospital ethics committee, with judicial scrutiny a last resort.[8]

Finally, McCormick reminds us again and again that treatment decisions for severely afflicted infants must be made within an *attitude of protection* of those most in need of our protection. "At stake, after all, is the life of a human being, and by consistent extension, the lives of many human beings. The moral fabric of a society can be gauged by the way it treats its most voiceless and voteless members" [49]. And the "pride" of the Judeo-Christian tradition is that "the weak and defenseless, the powerless and the unwanted, those whose grasp on the goods of life is most fragile . . . are cherished and protected as our neighbor in greatest need" ([38], p. 351). Any other attitude would be but a "racism of the adult world," at odds with the gospel and eventually corrosive of our humanity.

McCormick's confidence that a "reasonable" judgement about an infant's quality of life can indeed be reached is a reflection of his theological-ethical methodology and the moral epistemology upon which it is based. So let us turn now to an examination of his method.

2. McCORMICK'S "MODERATE TELEOLOGY"

In 1970, McCormick predicted that "[t]he next decade will be the era of value ethics. This term refers to an ethic whose chief preoccupation is with the goods and goals law is meant to achieve, institutions are meant to protect and promote and actions are meant to incarnate rather than with laws, institutions and external actions themselves" [31]. McCormick himself has gone a great way toward presenting a coherent, articulate and compelling model of value ethics.

He is not a 'rationalist' in the sense of claiming that moral convictions are predicated or discovered by reason alone. Instead, he sees reflective analysis as "an attempt to reinforce rationally, communicably, and from other sources what we grasp at a different level." We begin our quest for an understanding of definite moral obligations by asking, "What are the goods or values man can seek, the values that define his human opportunity, his flourishing?" ([38], p. 5; also [40], p. 313). And the answer is to be found in an examination of our "basic tendencies" (*inclinationes naturales* in the Thomistic tradition). What are these basic tendencies? McCormick lists at least the following as "basic inclinations present prior to acculturation":

... the tendency to preserve life; the tendency to mate and raise children; the tendency to seek out other men and obtain their approval – friendship; the tendency to establish good relations with unknown higher powers; the tendency to use intelligence in guiding action; the tendency to develop skills and exercise them in play and the fine arts ([40], p. 313; [38], p. 5).

From these inclinations we form "spontaneously and without reflection" basic principles of practical moral reasoning.

These inclinations, McCormick tells us, constitute our basic *values*; and we determine the morality of our conduct by how adequately "open" we are to these values, since each of them has its self-evident appeal "as a participation in the unconditioned Good we call God." In our lives one with another, realizing these values is "the only adequate way to love and attain God."

Basic values, together with "middle axioms" (or "mediating principles," derived from rational reflection on those values for application in concrete moral choices) comprise the "natural law." McCormick admits that our perception and grasp of basic human values are culturally qualified, or "shaped by our whole way of looking at the world." The 'distinctiveness' of *Christian* ethics lies in the Christian tradition's "illumination" of human values and its provision of a particular world-view, not in any material addition by Christianity to the moral norms rationally available to everyone. In other words,

... there is a *material* identity between Christian moral demands and those perceivable by reason. Whatever is distinct about Christian morality is found essentially in the style of life, the manner of accomplishing the moral tasks common to all men, not in the tasks themselves. Christian morality is, in its concreteness and materiality, *human* morality . . . The experience of Jesus is regarded as normative because he is believed to have experienced what it is to be *human* in the fullest way and at the deepest level. Christian ethics does not and cannot add to human ethical self-understanding as such any material content that is, in principle, strange or foreign to man as he exists and experiences himself ([38], p. 9).

Herein, too, is the core meaning of "reason informed by faith"; for that phrase does *not* mean, as McCormick is quick to point out, "reason *replaced* by faith" ([38], p. 10).

Sensitive, loving people might, of course, disagree on a particular value judgement. In McCormick's view, reflection on one's own *personal* experience is certainly one ingredient in an adequate theological ethics; but another is the aid provided by social and behavioral sciences ([39], p. 370). And, of course, we learn and have our consciences formed within a *community*. He suggests, further, that we might also 'test' in a rational way the value assessments which are implicit in our choices, and that we might establish "preference principles" for such tests. He offers (following Hans Reiner) examples of what these preference principles for assessing value-judgements might look like:

(1) Other things being equal, a non-postponable value is to be preferred to a postponable one.
(2) In conflict situations we must give preference to the lower but more 'foundational' value, even while continuing to acknowledge the higher as higher. For instance, we must feed a starving man before trying to preach the good news of salvation to him.
(3) Other things being equal, the common good is to be preferred to the good of the individual. Obviously, great sensitivity and discernment are needed here to avoid a crushing collectivism.
(4) Other things being equal, we should undertake tasks for which we are better suited than ones for which we are not.
(5) Other things being equal, we should prefer the good of those with a special relationship to our responsibility ([39], p. 369f.).

Because of the "illumination" of truly 'human' values afforded by the Christian tradition, this "sifting" or "sorting" of our experience through preference principles should be done in "an atmosphere highly charged with Christian intentionalities" (e.g., "the cruciform spirit of Christian life, resurrection destiny, the eschatological kingdom, the following of the poor and humble Christ") ([39], p. 370).

If the morality of our acts is determined, as suggested above, by our "openness" to basic values (prediscursively perceived), then just what does "openness" to them mean? McCormick suggests that it means: (1) always taking these values into account in our choices; (2) avoiding acting in ways that inhibit them and preferring ways that realize them (when we can); (3) making "an effort on their behalf when their realization in another is in extreme peril"; and (4) never choosing against a basic good (or 'value' – McCormick uses the two terms synonymously) ([40], p. 314). But now, of course, the crucial question becomes, What does it mean to "choose against a basic good?" (We have seen in Section 1, for example, that McCormick does not consider some choices against life-preserving medical treatment to be choices against a basic good.) McCormick's answer to this question – a rather involved answer – is what makes his method so distinctive and is also what has led some to charge him with being a thoroughgoing consequentialist (a matter to which we will return in Section 5 of this chapter). For, he holds that we perceive not just 'values' in general, but a hierarchy of goods (the *ordo bonorum*), and that moral choice involves preference for some values over others: morally correct actions realize the highest good available in the situation of choice. Our rationally-derived moral norms generally require or prohibit actions insofar as those actions affirm or deny values in the *ordo bonorum*. 'Exceptions' to moral norms apply where a value to be realized conflicts with an equal or greater value.

In order to understand McCormick's theory of values as a normative moral theory, we need some understanding of how it deals with decision-making in moral conflicts – that is, in those situations where choosing to act so as to realize one value will at the same time entail acting against another value. The notion of "preference principles" for weighing values may be useful to some extent. But a theory of values is put to the test, so to speak, when values which we hold to be *equally basic* or foundational come into conflict. The tradition of Catholic moral theology has produced – and McCormick has spent many years reflecting upon and revising – another sort of principle for determining moral obligation in choices of irreducible, basic value-conflict: the principle of the double effect.

This principle presupposes, as its name implies, that some particular actions may produce two effects, one good (affirming a value) and one evil (inhibiting a value). According to the traditional interpretation, such actions may be permitted if four conditions are met. First, the action itself, considered independently of its effects, must not be morally evil. This criterion has historically excluded at the outset some actions considered intrinsically evil, such as perjury, blasphemy, masturbation and murder. Second, the agent must directly *intend* only the good effect; he/she may only *permit* the evil effect (although both are foreseen). Third, the evil effect must not be the *means* by which the good effect is produced (for a good end cannot justify the use of morally evil means). And fourth, there must be a *proportionate reason* for the action despite its evil effect. That is, the good to be produced must be seen to compensate for or exceed the tolerated evil effect (Cf., e.g., [28], p. 13).

Perhaps the best-known medical application of the principle of the double effect is in the issue of abortion. In the Church's view, 'abortion' means the direct killing of an unborn person and is always wrong. But in two specific sorts of cases "justifiable fetal death" may be allowed by application of the double-effect principle: ectopic (tubal) pregnancies and pregnancies involving a cancerous uterus. In these cases the action under consideration – removal of a pathological organ – is not an evil in itself. The surgeon's direct *intent* is to save the mother's life; the foreseeable demise of the fetus within the removed organ is merely permitted. Further, fetal death follows from the life-saving surgery and is not the *means* to preserving the mother's life (while any direct evacuation of a normal uterus would constitute unjustifiable abortion). Finally, there is a proportionate reason for the surgery, inasmuch as it preserves maternal life and forgoing it would predictably mean death for both mother and fetus.

McCormick is among a number of Catholic moral theologians who have criticized the traditional understanding of double effect on one or more of its conditions. In his attempts to revise the traditional view he has stressed the interpretive primacy of "proportionate reason" as the key to justifying actions with predictably mixed consequences. And proportionate reason means more than mere quantitative weighing of consequences (as it might appear in the above example of justifying one fetal death in part by balancing it against the probable deaths of both mother and fetus). Proportionate reason means, for McCormick, an analysis of all circumstances surrounding an action (or omission) which determine its qualitative moral *meaning*.

Seen in this light, determination of the meaning of an action must logically precede any determination of whether the action itself constitutes an "intrinsic moral evil." So McCormick parts company with those traditional categorizations of intrinsically evil actions which underlie the first condition of the double effect principle. Instead, he begins with another traditionally-accepted distinction: *physical* evil vs. *moral* evil.[9] A physical (or "premoral") evil is an objective disvalue (e.g., wounding, killing, deception), but may be justified for an adequate (proportionate) reason – e.g., in self-defense, protection of the innocent, etc. A moral evil (or *sin*) is a physical evil perpetrated disproportionately or frivolously. Dishonesty, injustice, murder, and infidelity are examples of *moral* evils and are forbidden by exceptionless moral norms – i.e., they are "intrinsic evils." However, as McCormick and others have pointed out, these terms describe more than simply an action considered by itself (see, e.g., [24], [27]). 'Murder,' for instance, specifies not only an act of killing but also the circumstances, object, and intention in the act – all of which have already been adjudged "disproportionate" by the employment of the term 'murder' itself. Just as every act which brings about death is not necessarily 'murder,' so are other premoral evils not necessarily moral evils. Of course, premoral evils are not *neutral* in themselves; without proportionate reason they are moral evils as well. But McCormick's point is that the designation "intrinsic moral evil" cannot consistently be premised upon a description of premoral evil alone but must result from a determination of the *meaning* of the act through proportionate reason.

We should note here, as McCormick himself does, that this notion of proportionate reason – of weighing "premoral" goods/evils in particular circumstances in order to determine "moral" good/evil – is conceptually similar to W.D. Ross's rule-deontological methodology. Ross holds that in many situations we face irreducible conflicts between "prima facie" (or presumptive) moral duties – e.g., "keep a promise to meet a friend for lunch" vs. "stop to help the injured victim of an accident" – and that we must weigh the relative importance of them in order to determine the most pressing, "actual" moral duty *in that situation* of choice. Ross's language is consistently that of duty-based right/wrong and not of value-based good/evil, but it seems clear to McCormick that if Ross's "actual" duty might be, e.g., *not* to keep a promise, then this can only mean "that a more urgent *good* is at stake in some way." For that is what a "duty more pressing" means, in McCormick's view. Thus, he sees close conceptual ties between his method of proportionate reasoning and Ross's method of weighing "prima facie" duties (see [37], p. 253f.; and [43]).

Another ramification of McCormick's method is that "exceptionless" moral norms do not (or should not) prohibit physical acts considered in the abstract; rather, they express a determination that the premoral evil in question cannot possibly have a proportionate reason and thus must be seen as a moral evil:

A behavioral norm is exceptionless only if it prescribes a value that cannot conflict with other values, or if it does, one that always deserves the preference. *Always deserves the preference* is but a way of saying that (at least in our perspective) it overrides the other value, is more urgent than the other value, or disallows feature-dependent exceptions. It is a way of saying that choice of the other value would be disproportionate, or, that there is not proportionate reason either thinkable or realistically imaginable for overriding the value ([37], p. 232).

As an example of such an exceptionless moral norm, McCormick cites approvingly Bruno Schuller's claim that we must never deliberately and intentionally cause others to do that which we – or they – conscientiously believe to be moral evil.[10] For, any person's moral integrity is itself a *moral* value – indeed, the highest value in life – and thus there could never be a proportionate reason for its sacrifice.

Now, although the physical evil/moral evil distinction (and the allowance of some physical evils for porportionate reasons) can be found within the Thomistic tradition of moral theology, the tradition has also *excluded* two categories of "intrinsically evil" actions from such a considerations: (1) actions *against nature* (i.e., certain sexual actions such as masturbation, contraception and sterilization); and, (2) actions that are wrong due to a *lack of right* (e.g., direct killing of the innocent or dissolution of a sacramental and consummated marriage). McCormick's reinterpretation of the double effect principle rejects both sorts of exclusion. For, in the latter category, the acts in question are already described *within particular contexts*; and the phrase "lack of right" itself indicates a qualification *based upon* proportionate reason – i.e., a judgement that this value cannot be outweighed by other values in this context. As for the former category, McCormick questions the logic of singling out these particular premoral evils (i.e., those inhering in sexual function) as absolute *moral* evils. If we claim, for example, that the premoral evil of sterilization is intrinsically (and absolutely) evil, then "we are attributing a value and an inviolability to the sexual endowment which tradition has refused to give life itself" ([39], p. 591). In short, consistency demands that we not claim "intrinsic moral evil" of any premoral evil in the abstract; rather, we must first judge its proportionality (in the *ordo bonorum*) vis-à-vis other concretely realizable values. And, further,

... when an action is always morally wrong, it is so not because of unnaturalness or defect of right (as recent tradition contends), but because *when taken as a whole*, the nonmoral evil outweighs the nonmoral good, and therefore the action is disproportionate ([39], p. 710).

Given this understanding of proportionate reason as determining the moral meaning of particular actions, the traditional category of absolutely forbidden premoral evils is virtually emptied and the first condition of double effect loses any independent significance. The second condition – that the agent directly intend only the good effect of his/her action – is also transformed from its traditional interpretation in McCormick's proportionalism. For, in his view, the requirement that a physical evil never be *directly* caused has no moral decisiveness as such. The heart of the matter is instead whether such evils are *intended* or only *permitted*. McCormick is persuaded by Bruno Schuller (see [56], [37]) that intending/permitting has meaning with reference to the agent's basic moral attitude of approval or disapproval of the caused evil. With respect to premoral evils, *intending* a caused evil as a means (of producing a proportionate good) and *permitting* that evil can both be consistent with the same attitude of *disapproval* of that evil: i.e., "I would not do this if there were any other choice . . ." (Of course, intending a premoral evil as an end in itself would entail *approval* of it and would be morally wrong.) Further, if one has judged that the good result of his action will outweigh the evil result, then is not his intentionality clearly and directly oriented toward producing the good effect? So, both permitting premoral evil and intending it as a means can pertain to moral disapproval of it, and both can be morally justifiable.

But when is an action that causes premoral evil *not* morally justifiable?

An action, like killing, is morally wrongful when it must be said to turn against a basic good. It is an action entailing an attitude of will, a mental attitude against a basic good (life); an attitude describable as approval of evil . . . This cannot be identified with intending the evil as a means (*direct* as traditionally understood . . .). It happens when (1) the evil is intended; or (2) when it is caused without necessity. When, however, it is reluctantly caused because necessary (whether permitted as a nonmeans, or intended as a means), it does not entail a bad moral will, or 'turning against a basic good' ([37], p. 261f.).

The term "necessary" here represents a key aspect of McCormick's notion of proportionate reason. Killing (to use the same example) is proportionate when it is "the *only way imaginable* to prevent greater loss of life" ([37], p. 262).

At this point we have touched upon McCormick's reformulation of the third and last remaining condition of double effect: that the evil effect must not be the means to producing the good effect. This condition is essentially meaningless in McCormick's view, since the *moral* evilness of any premoral evil effect must be determined by proportionate reason, which involves choosing the lesser of unavoidable premoral evils and not willing any evil as an end in itself. What *is* meaningful for McCormick, however, is the condition that a premoral evil means must be a *causally necessary* means to the higher good; the evil result must be of a piece with the only conceivable means of producing the least harmful overall outcome in the circumstance. This limits the extent to which "proportionalism" can be seen to be simply a balancing of predicted consequences. McCormick often points to the difference himself by referring to the so-called "Caiaphas principle" in utilitarian moral philosophy – that is, that one may be justified in sacrificing one innocent person to save many. One well-worn example of this principle is the hypothethical case of a Southern sheriff or judge who believes he can prevent many lethal consequences of a violent lynch mob by framing one black suspect (who he knows to be innocent) on a rape charge.[11] While some consequentialists have seen this as a simple lose-one-save-many situation, it is not "proportionate" (for McCormick) in that there is no inherent link between the killing of the innocent suspect and the preservation of other lives. To believe that there is would be to reject the value of (the mob's) free will for doing good or evil. The sheriff would not be choosing the proportionate "lesser evil."

In contrast to this example of disproportionate and morally wrong sacrifice of life, McCormick also frequently points to the (fortunately rare) abortion dilemma in which a physician must either abort a fetus to save the mother (e.g., if she requires abdominal surgery to correct a life-threatening aneurysm located behind the uterus) or else not abort and let the mother and child die. According to the traditional interpretation of double effect, the physician must not operate because (s)he would be *killing an innocent* with *direct intent* as a *means* to saving the mother. But McCormick would hold such an abortive measure to be the proportionate "lesser evil" in such circumstance, *not* because it is a simple, predictable save-one-or-lose-two dilemma but because it is concretely possible to affirm the value of at least one life in this case and because the abortive surgery is "intrinsically and inescapably connected" with doing so.

Thus, the criterion of necessity places a significant restraint upon judgements of "proportionate" sacrifice of premoral value. Moreover, McCormick suggests that a lack of necessity also means that the value being sought – the 'higher good' – may in fact be *undermined* by the action in question. He develops this idea through the notion of "associated basic goods." Specifically, he holds that some basic goods in the *ordo bonorum* are certainly interrelated (or "associated") with one another such that injury to one of them involves injury to the others associated with it. And value-sacrifice which is efficacious but not "essentially connected" (necessary) to the preservation of another value may therefore entail sacrifice of other values "associated" with the value sought (and thus injury to the latter).

This is a complicated concept, and one which demands concrete illustration for its clarification. One of the examples McCormick employs is Joseph Fletcher's case of Mrs. Bergmeier, the post-war German internee in a Russian work camp who allowed a "friendly" camp guard to impregnate her in order to effect her release (as a medical liability) and return to her distraught family. Mrs. Bergmeier's action is perhaps "factually efficacious" in McCormick's view, but certainly not causally *necessary* for preserving the value of her freedom. For, her captors are themselves free to change their minds and release her at any time. But her action implicitly asserts that her captors will end her unjust captivity only if she yields sexually and becomes pregnant – that is, she is expressing a necessary causal connection between her action and their response. Because there is *not* such a necessary connection, her choice "to yield to extortion" is also "to deny the extortioner's liberty" (as well as denying the good of conjugal sexuality in marriage) to choose the right for himself. And, "since liberty is a basic value, to assault it is to assualt these others, too" ([37], p. 239). In this case, denial of the guard's moral freedom is essentially a denial of the very value – liberty – Mrs. Bergmeier seeks. Her choice is, in McCormick's view, disproportionate.

Another, similar example is that of obliteration bombing in wartime in order to shorten the war and thus avoid many future casualties (e.g., Allied bombing of Hamburg, Dresden, Hiroshima, etc.). This understanding of proportion is wrong, McCormick tells us, even if the war aims of the bombing nation (such as resisting unjust aggression and preserving political freedoms) are just. It is wrong because counter-people warfare undermines, through the association of goods, the value it seeks to preserve:

Making innocent (noncombatant) persons the object of our targeting is a form of extortion in international affairs that contains an implicit denial of human freedom. Human freedom is undermined when extortionary actions are accepted and elevated and universalized. Because such freedom is an associated good upon which the very good of life heavily depends, undermining it in the manner of my defense of life is undermining life itself– is disprotionate ([37], p. 236).

Furthermore, denial of the value of the enemy's freedom and responsibility also denies the value of our own. And our subsequent deliberations and decisions will reflect this disproportionate denial of value:

> Is anyone willing to assert confidently that there is no connection between Nagasaki-Hiroshima and the senseless slaughters that occurred in South Vietnam? Once the manner of our protection of a basic good reduces or removes by implication the basis for rational limitation of violence (liberty), then irrational (disproportionate) things are going to happen. These irrational things point back to and reveal the disproportion in our original responses ([37], p. 238).

These comments reflect one other feature of McCormick's proportionalism to which we should attend. In some of the examples cited so far, the 'premoral' evils mentioned have been, literally and descriptively, 'physical' evils – e.g., killing, sterilization, masturbation, and so on. But as the above discussion of associated goods makes clear, the values we protect or sacrifice are not always tangible, clearly measurable entities in our 'physical' milieu. Political extortion's "implicit denial of human freedom," for example, has to do not so much with the quantifiable consequence of restrained activity, but rather with a qualitative disrespect for the very notion of responsible human free-choice within the express action of extortion itself. In another example – that of a voter whose candidate is a sure winner and who sees more utility in staying home on election day – McCormick cites the value of "expression of solidarity" in an action (voting) which might appear quantitatively useless. The upshot of all this is that "proportionate reason" cannot be limited in its scope to a mere assessment of physical harms visited upon persons or property as a consequence of value-sacrifice, or of such harms as the definition of value-sacrifice. Proportionate reasons must also consider 'symbolic' or 'expressive' harms – harms to values which exist for us as abstract notions such as "community" or "freedom of the will." Certainly it is more difficult to 'weigh' values of this sort than it is to assess the relative value-sacrifice in, say, losing a hand vs. losing one's life. But such conceptual values form the fabric of the moral or spiritual self; so erosion of one's commitment to these values entails a threat to the self's moral/spiritual integrity. And, since that integrity is our highest good in life, any threat to it must be considered very seriously.

We have seen in this section that the key to understanding McCormick's ethical method as it relates to value-conflict resolution is his notion of proportionate reason. To summarize, proportionate reason demands that in conflict situations we should always choose to protect the higher value in the *ordo bonorum*. When equally basic values are at stake and protection of one of them entails sacrifice of the other, then such a sacrifice can be proportionate if and only if it is the only way to avoid even greater destruction of value – that is, if it is *necessary* for the preservation of those basic goods which can be preserved. Finally, proportionate reason requires that our judgements of 'necessity' in such circumstances be tempered with an unwillingness to choose means of protecting basic goods which might in fact threaten those goods by injuring other, associated goods.

Clearly the *ordo bonorum* represents for McCormick a more-or-less objective system of values for whose protection we are morally responsible. Human life is a basic value; human freedom of self-determination is another. But it would seem that there are situations in which an individual, in the process of exercising his/her free self-determination, chooses to act without proportionate reason – that is, to act against a basic good such as life itself – as viewed by other persons. What should the community's response be in such conflicts of valuation? The next section will examine McCormick's approach to this question in terms of the issue of 'autonomous' refusals of life-preserving medical treatment.

3. VALUES, COMMUNITY AND AUTONOMY: McCORMICK AND TREATMENT REFUSALS

One of the most frequently addressed issues in medical ethics over the past two decades has been the conflict between patient autonomy and professional paternalism. The literature is filled with actual and hypothetical case-studies in which patients' own decisions about their treatment (quite often decisions to end their treatment) are ignored or overridden by professionals' decisions to 'help' the patient by continuing or expanding treatment. The notion of 'paternalism' (or 'parentalism') involves the assumption that person A is making choices *for* person B without B's behest or voluntary consent, and that A is seeking to promote what (s)he believes to be in B's 'best interests' in doing so.[12] The major philosophical criticism of paternalism is that it shows a lack of respect for person B by depriving B of self-determination with respect to his/her body and personal future; the freedom of such self-determination, it is argued, is demanded by the principle of autonomy (as a manifestation of 'respect for persons').

Arguments for respecting a patient's 'right' to self-determination generally presuppose that individuals have differing sets of personal goals, commitments, religious beliefs, etc., and that every rational person is best situated to recognize his/her own best interests based upon his/her own personal goals/values. So, respecting the patient's autonomy entails respecting his/her own self-chosen ends because they are self-chosen. Medical paternalism, on the other hand, involves choosing goals (of treatment) for the patient on the assumption that the patient's self-defined best interests will be (or *should* be) congruent with the care-giver's definition of those interests. It is because those definitions are *not* always congruent that medical paternalism becomes a practical moral problem.

Those who argue in favor of admitting exceptions to our duty to respect the claim of patient autonomy attempt to justify paternalistic interventions on either of two bases: (1) because the *patient* is incompetent, irrational, or otherwise incapable of determining his/her own best interests and making choices thereon (and thus stands in peril of choosing what will be harmful to him/her); or (2) because the *substance* of what the patient chooses for himself/herself is seen to be unreasonably self-harming (on some ostensibly objective scale of 'reasonable' best interests), even though the patient's rational powers do not appear limited or encumbered. The former argument seeks to justify cases of what has been called "weak" paternalism, so named because it questions not the *right* of self-determination but rather the *capacity* or *competence* of some persons to choose and act autonomously. The latter argument would support overriding autonomous self-regarding choices by competent persons, and thus has been termed "strong" paternalism.[13]

Now, we have seen that McCormick's moral theory emphasizes values to be realized; moral duties and rights are derived from the values they tend to support. In this perspective, the moral right of self-determination reflects the value of human freedom and responsibility. But that value, and therefore that right, are "conditional" and limited by other values (see, e.g., [40], p. 319f.; [47], p. 1132f.). As a result, McCormick would defend some treatment interventions which would fit the above description of "strong" paternalism.

The issue of life-preserving medical treatment and patient acceptance/rejection of it is addressed by McCormick in a 1976 article, "The Moral Right to Privacy" ([38], pp. 352–61). In his view, the Catholic moral tradition has consistently dealt with the right of self-determination in health care in terms of the (limited) *duty* of preservation of life. (Some of the limitations on the duty to preserve life have been reviewed in Section 1, above.) Since the individual patient has the best knowledge of what may be called a 'reasonable benefit' or an 'unreasonable burden' to him/her, (s)he has the *right* to "those means that make personal execution of this duty possible, and to those means that best provide for the practical admission of limits on this duty" ([38], p. 358). Self-determination is, in this regard, a necessary means to the fulfillment of personal duty. The supposition in all of this is that self-determination of treatment serves the "best over-all good of patients"; so, self-determination is a "conditional" or "instrumental" good – a good "precisely insofar as it is the instrument whereby the best interest of the patient are served by it" ([38], p. 359).

McCormick goes on to point out two limitations on the right of self-determination which follow from this interpretation. First, the very *reason* for the right disappears when its exercise "is *de facto* and in the circumstances no longer to the overall good of the person involved." If, for example, a patient wishes to exercise self-determination "in a way commonly regarded as destructive to self" – suicide – then the right is no longer supported by its underlying good. Second, the right to self-determination says nothing about its exercise to the detriment of others; it is rooted solely in the best interests of the individual in question ([38], p. 359).

Clearly, the central and dominant notion here is the patient's 'best interests.' The moral right of self-determination exists, we are told, because it is a necessary means to insuring that patients' best interests will be served. But we are also told that an individual's exercise of self-determination does not always or necessarily produce choices coincident with what his/her best interests actually are. In such cases, intervention by another is morally warranted in order to protect the patient's actual best interests.

Stated abstractly, the process of recognizing and protecting one's own best interests is nothing more or less than recognizing self-referential values in the objective order of goods (*ordo bonorum*) and applying proportionate reason in self-referential choices. In this light, 'suicide' amounts to any choice against preserving one's own life which is not proportionate. As for determining whether a particular rejection of life-preserving medical treatment might *be* proportionate, the framework for judgement is objectively the same as for third-party treatment decisions (for infants or incompetents): the factors involved are the *uselessness* of available treatment and/or the *burdensomeness* of accepting that treatment. Applied to the cases of persons with terminal illnesses, McCormick suggests a broad latitude of "reasonable" (and morally proportionate) self-interpretations of "burdensomeness" while at the same time admitting that some interpretations will be unreasonable (and should invite intervention):

... [T]he appropriate mix of values during dying, how one shall live while dying, belongs to the patient. And here patients may and do differ within the range of morally acceptable options.

Of the three key values present (preservation of life, human freedom, lack of pain), some will choose to maximize freedom, others to minimize pain even with the diminution of freedom. Still others will manage their dying with a controlling view of the financial and/or psychological condition of their dear ones ... Treatment that conforms to such wishes and perspectives may be considered reasonable (morally appropriate), always allowing for legal appeal by physician or hospital if a patient is judged to be *frivolously jeopardizing life* ([38], p. 399f.)

There are, then, plural values which in McCormick's view might offer proportionate reason for a terminally ill person's acceptance *or* rejection of life-prolonging treatment; there are also non-proportional values whose preference would be "frivolous" and whose choice would warrant paternalistic intervention. We are given few specifics as to exactly *which* choices against continuing treatment would constitute frivolous jeopardizations of life.[14] But McCormick is confident that rational onlookers will recognize those disproportionate choices and that they will approve of paternalism in order to override them in favor of the patient's actual best interests:

Most people ... would think that what is actually in a person's best interests ought to prevail over what the deluded or misguided person thinks is in his best interests. In this sense ...

most people would be objective or normative in determining best interests, for best interests are best interests, not putative best interests ([38], p. 107).

Underlying McCormick's claims about the proper limits of self-determination is a more foundational claim about the notion of proportionate reason itself – namely, that one cannot claim "that a reason is truly proportionate *because a particular individual thinks so*" or that the determination of proportionality is "the exclusive prerogative of the individual" ([39], p. 699). Of course, a reason is not truly proportionate simply because "most people" think so, either. We learn and form our consciences within a community of persons, and communities can ignore or misplace values just as individuals can. But McCormick stresses again and again that "individualism" cannot be the path to comprehension and protection of moral values. For, "[t]he preference principles which attempt to sort out the claims of the *ordo bonorum* . . . are the result of common reflection and discourse" – activities in and for the community ([39], p. 699). This implies not that the community's values will always be objectively correct but certainly that "a realistic individual will understand the dangers of trying to discover moral truth alone, of deciding what is right and wrong in isolation from a pool of wisdom and reflection far greater than the individual's" ([39], p. 768).

To summarize, then, one of the moral purposes of communities is to inform, nurture, and sometimes correct the determinations of proportionate reason which individuals must make. Individual self-determination is a *bonum utile* (instrumental good) existing both within and alongside the broader *bonum utile* of community reflection and discernment – both of which are in the service of those objective goods which define our 'best interests.'

The relationship between individual and community has been considered in this section with reference to defining and acting toward the individual's good ("best interests") alone. But another sort of moral relationship between individual and community also finds characteristic expression in McCormick's theological ethics: the obligations of individuals toward the best interests of others in the community. The next section will deal with a concrete application of those obligations.

4. GOODS OF SELF AND GOODS OF OTHERS: McCORMICK ON EXPERIMENTATION WITH CHILDREN

The requirement of voluntary, informed consent of all subjects in medical research has been recognized almost universally, at least since its articulation nearly 50 years ago at the Nuremburg "Doctors' Trials." But whether that requirement categorically and unexceptionably excludes all potential subjects who are not competent to consent has been a matter of much debate. Is it ever morally acceptable for a parent or guardian to give a 'proxy' or vicarious consent for research participation by a minor child or an incompetent person? In attempting to answer that question in particular cases, the courts (and quite a few physicians, philosophers, and theologians) have focused upon what has been called the "substituted judgement" standard of consent. The doctrine of substituted judgement requires that a guardian make decisions for an incompetent or not-yet-competent person on the basis of the best the guardian can know of that person's best interests and personal preferences. In other words, a proper substituted judgement is one which we are confident the incompetent person *would* make if competent to make it. In the case of children, whose personal preferences for or against consent cannot yet be surmised, substituted judgement amounts to a "reasonable presumption" of what the child would want; this presumption is usually based upon whether the treatment or research in question might provide some therapeutic benefit for that child. Thus, for example, proxy consent for a child's participation in therapeutic research – that is, experimentation designed to produce information useful both in treating future patients *and* in treating (or preventing) illness in the experimental subjects themselves – is often accepted as morally licit because the child-subject could be presumed reasonably to want the medical benefit for himself/herself. On the same grounds, though, substituted judgement would not validate proxy consent for a child's participation in nontherapeutic research, since that experimentation is by definition oriented toward producing data useful in treating other, future patients while offering no therapeutic benefit to its experimental subjects.

McCormick believes that consent is indeed "at the heart of the matter" of experimentation, for it would be morally wrong to treat children or anybody else as mere "objects" of research. And he believes that valid parental consent must be based upon "a construction of what the child would wish could he consent for himself." However, he also believes, on the basis of the natural law theory of values he has articulated, that a construction of the child's wishes should take into account more than simply the prospect of therapeutic benefit. A child *would*, he argues, generally choose the goods of self-preservation and health because he *ought* to; such choices are proportionate value choices. But, he asks, are there *other* things "that the child *ought*, as a human being, to choose precisely because and insofar as they are goods definitive of his growth and flourishing?" And his answer is affirmative:

To pursue the good that is human life means not only to choose and support this value in one's own case, but also in the case of others when the opportunity arises. In other words, the individual *ought* also to take into account, realize, and make efforts in behalf of the lives of others also, for we are social beings, and the goods that define our growth and invite to it are goods that reside also in others. It can be good for one to pursue and support this good in others. Therefore, when it factually is good, we may say that one *ought* to do so (as opposed to not doing so). If this is true of all of us up to a point and within limits, it is no less true of the infant. He would choose to do so because he *ought* to do so ([38], p. 62).

Now, two immediate question are raised by this statement of the matter. First, what is McCormick claiming about the moral agency of infants and young children in his use of the word "ought"? And, second, what does he mean by proposing that this "ought" exists "up to a point and within limits" – particularly in the concrete situation of non-therapeutic research?

As for his use of ought-language, McCormick argues that he is not treating the infant as an adult by implying or imputing moral agency and moral obligation. His language of 'ought' need not imply actual obligations. "It is," he writes, "simply a device, a construction (as is also the language of what the infant *would* choose) to get at the reasonableness of our expectations and interventions" ([38], p. 90). For if we expect of *adults* a (limited) willingness to seek the good of others, it is not *because* they are adults that we expect it, but because they are *social persons* and we expect they will recognize and respond to the claims rooted in their natural sociality. Applying the language of 'ought' to infants is McCormick's way of highlighting the fact that his focus is on the good of sociality, not age, and "this sociality is shared quite as much by infants as by adults" ([38], p. 90).

As for the "limits" of what we ought to do for others' good, McCormick is quick to distinguish between the entailments of the good of sociality and those of the "good of expressed charity." If an adult person should choose to promote the good of others by donating an organ, for example, or by participating in research which involves risk, pain or inconvenience, then he may be affirming his sociality in doing so. But in accepting those risks he has gone beyond the 'ought' of sharing the burden of promoting others' good implied by his natural sociality; he is instead expressing charity. No one else can reasonably *presume* his consent to such risky actions for two reasons. First, whether the acceptance of risk would be personally (subjectively) good for the individual is a "highly individual affair"; only he can know if it is proportionate with respect to his own commitments, responsibilities, plans, etc. Second, and more importantly, these risk-accepting actions become human goods for the donor or subject "precisely because and therefore only when they are voluntary, for the personal good under discussion is the good of expressed charity" ([38], p. 63).

By analogy to situations of proxy consent for children, we could never presume that a child would consent to any risk-involving nontherapeutic measure. What we may presume, however, in McCormick's judgement, is that a child would be (because he *ought* to be) willing to "share in the general effort and burden of health maintenance and disease control [which] is part of our flourishing and growth as humans" when that sharing does not entail real personal risk ([38], p. 62). These proxy choices do not pertain to charity, but rather "pertain to the area of social justice, one's personal bearing of his share of the burden that all may flourish and prosper" ([38], p. 67). In concrete terms, McCormick believes that a child ought to, and thus would, consent to participation in non-therapeutic research that holds promise of considerable benefit to other children and that would involve for him/her "no discernible risks, no notable pain, [and] no notable inconvenience." The experimentation should also be well-designed scientifically, so as to offer genuine hope of producing beneficial knowledge, and it should be a last and necessary resort which cannot succeed unless the subjects are children (as opposed to adults or lab animals) ([38], p. 64).

McCormick admits that the notion of "no discernible risk" can be somewhat "slippery." It is rendered somewhat more slippery by his occasional replacement of that phrase with "no notable risk" and even "minimal risk." These are not fully synonymous expressions, and Paul Ramsey suggests that they denote an "accordion" guideline of uncertain limits ([55], pp. 21–30). At any rate, McCormick allows that "discernible risk" and "undue discomfort" certainly involve value judgements which are the responsibility of the medical profession to make. Further, he agrees with at least the rationale behind Ramsey's criticism of "accordion" terminology. For, Ramsey's concern is that adjectives like "notable" or "minimal" might be construed as implying a calculus or ratio in which the subject's risk is *compared* to the extent of expected benefit to others. And McCormick insists that a risk/benefit ratio of this type is unacceptable. "Low risk" to the subject must be assessed independently from all other considerations and must mean, in human judgement and for all practical purposes, "no realistic risk." If it is interpreted in any other way, "it opens the door wide to a utilitarian subordination of the individual to the collectivity. It goes beyond what individuals would want because they *ought* to" ([38], p. 65).

Moreover, our assessments of "no realistic risk," and thus our presumptions of what a noncompetent child *ought* to choose, must also be subject to modification based upon the individual child's particular circumstances. McCormick cites the special consideration demanded by institutionalized children as an example. Medical history shows that we have been tempted to regard these children as "lesser human beings" with regard to the risks we will subject them to; that their institutionalization makes them a controllable group, and thus tempting research subjects; and that experimentation on them has been relatively less exposed to public scrutiny than that involving other groups of children. For all these reasons, they may be in danger of our overstepping the boundary of "no discernible risk" and presuming for them more than we all ought to want. And the institutionalized child "need not *ought to want* if this involves him in real dangers of going beyond this point" ([38], p. 69).

In a sense, McCormick's view of proper proxy consent moves beyond the usual limitations of a "substituted judgement" standard to include a further, "reasonable person" standard. His version does not wholly *supplant* the former with the latter; what the child *would choose* remains a part of his focus. But he has broadened the basis of presumption by offering reasons *why* the child *ought* to, and therefore would, so choose founded upon reasonable expression of the child's own good of sociality. Of course, since this good is constitutive of all of us as social human beings, it follows that what a child ought to consent to is what we all ought to consent to. And if we adults are not willing to "bear our fair share that all may prosper," then certainly we must reexamine our attitudes toward, and consents for, children. "Otherwise, we are practicing a racism of the adult world" [35].

As a 'postscript' to this section, then, we should note that in McCormick's view our minimal social 'ought' might conceivably outweigh a lack of voluntariness (for non-risky research) among individuals who *are competent* to consent for themselves. In his own words,

> Even though it can be argued that we all have duties in this area [research], duties of readiness and willingness, it is understandable, even desirable, that informed consent accompany the fulfillment of these duties. For consensual community is something to be promoted wherever possible. If, however, not enough volunteers are available for minimal risk experimentation and the research seems to be of overriding importance to the public health, it would not be unjust of the government to recruit experimental subjects, for example, by lottery, just as it is not unjust for government to draft soldiers for national self-defense. But just as a volunteer army is preferable, if adequate, to a drafted one, so are volunteer experimental subjects. Could they speak to the point, this is what children . . . would probably be telling us [35].

5. PROPORTIONATE REASON AND CONSEQUENTIALISM

The moral theory presented in this chapter is clearly value-dominant in the sense that moral obligation is determined by rational assessment of which actions or rules of practice will protect the highest values in an objective, "prediscursively perceived" hierarchy of values. So, as we have seen, assessment of the consequences of actions (or rules) is an essential feature of "proportionate reason." The question with which we will conclude this chapter, then, is this: To what extent does McCormick's teleological theory represent a genuinely "consequentialist" morality?

Several of McCormick's critics, including both theological ethicists and moral philosophers, have described his ethical method as consequentalist or utilitarian in stripe.[15] Frederick Carney maintains, for instance, that proportionate reason is "unquestionably a form of utilitarianism" in that it focuses upon weighing values (in the *ordo bonorum*) in a "calculus." Further, the value theory upon which it is constructed bears similarities to what has been called "ideal utilitarianism" ([10], pp. 93, 97f.). Germain Grisez refers to McCormick as a consequentialist (by which he means one who holds that defining 'right' and 'wrong' depends upon "efficiency in promoting measurable good results") and goes on to label consequentialist moral theory as "incomprehensible" and "dangerous nonsense" ([25], pp. 24, 27). John Connery identifies "proportionalism" with "consequentialism" in that both deny "the possibility of an independent morality deriving from the object of the act" ([14], p. 234 n. 4). The proportionalist has to admit, in Connery's view, that "the end really justifies the means" ([14], p. 276). And as a result of the influence of proportionalism, he argues, the norms governing some acts (like extra-marital sex) "become exposed to exception-making in a way that can be very subjective and arbitrary" ([15], p. 495). Alasdair MacIntyre agrees that McCormick's method allows too broad a scope to notions of proportion and weighing of values, and concludes that because "his teleology lacks the necessary complexity, he slides toward and possibly into consequentialism" ([50], p. 438). William Frankena is – astonishingly – somewhat unsure as to which of his many categories of ethical theory McCormick's fits into, but finds that "on the basis of what we have seen *thus far* I see no alternative but to interpret McCormick as a utilitarian of some sort . . ." ([23], p. 159). James Childress offers a more modest (and more specific) claim; he is willing to agree with McCormick's own claims that the latter's perspective is *not* utilitarian, but insists nonetheless that "it does share some important structural similarities and problems with rule-utilitarianism" ([11], p. 41).

In attempting any assessment of such claims, we must of course also attend to the *meaning* of key terms like 'teleology,' 'consequentialism,' and 'utilitarianism.'

Teleology: The term 'teleology' was first paired and contrasted with 'deontology' by C.D. Broad in 1930 to provide a typology of theories of moral obligation. According to Broad, deontological theories (from the Greek *deon*, duty) "hold that there are ethical propositions of the form: 'Such and such a kind of action would always be right (or wrong) in such and such circumstances, no matter what its consequences might be.'" On the other hand, teleological theories (from the Greek *telos*, 'end' or 'goal') hold that "the rightness or wrongness of an action is always determined by its tendency to produce consequences which are intrinsically good or bad" ([5], p. 206f.). More recently, William Frankena has altered Broad's distinction slightly to define teleology as making consequences the "one and only . . . ultimate right-making characteristic" and to define deontology as allowing "that there are other considerations that may make an action or rule right or obligatory besides the goodness or badness of its consequences . . ." ([22], pp. 14ff.). Note that Frankena, a professed deontologist, defines 'deontology' more inclusively (with respect to possible right-making characteristics) than does Broad (who seems to lean toward teleology); and Frankena's definition of 'teleology' appears more exclusive, or narrow, than Broad's. Lisa Cahill suggests that these nuances of definition represent a tendency among moral philosophers and theologians to define their own preferred theory as the more comprehensive and capable of considering both the intrinsic character of actions and their consequences.[16] Perhaps this is because both 'sides' have observed, with W.D. Ross, that "both the notion of the right and the notion of the good are implied in the study of moral questions, and any one who tries to work with one only will sooner or later find himself forced to introduce the other."[17] Moreover, those of us who have applied typological zeal to fitting various moral theories into Broad's two categories should not lose sight of his own original caveat:

> We must remember . . . that *purely* deontological and *purely* teleological theories are rather ideal limits than real existents. Most actual theories are mixed, some being predominantly deontological and others predominantly teleological ([5], p. 207f.).

This observation is particularly germane, in my view, to any fair examination of McCormick's moral theory. For, some of his critics seem to be attributing to him (and then attacking) a notion of 'pure' teleology much like that defined by Frankena, while McCormick describes himself as a "moderate teleologist," by which he means one who insists "that other elements than consequences function in moral rightness and wrongness" ([37], pp. 200, 245). (This description of "moderate teleology" bears a striking resemblance to Frankena's definition of *deontology* above!) Exactly *how* elements other than consequences function in McCormick's theory will receive further scrutiny below.

These comments about teleology have thus far been limited to a particular sort of teleology, namely, a teleology of moral obligation which focuses upon the results of actions. But inasmuch as 'teleology' is definitionally concerned with discourse about ends (*teloi*), other teleologies organize and account for various realms of ends (e.g., the ends of personal virtue, of human nature, or of institutions). Aristotle defined the *telos* of human persons as virtue or excellence, and organized a notion of morality around the realization of that end. Thomas Aquinas expounded a teleology of nature and of human persons which included both natural and supernatural ends for human beings. Man's final *telos*, in Thomas's view, is *beatitudo* (happiness with God), for which he believed all persons have an innate desire. "Natural" *teloi* are ordained in creation as themselves means toward this final end. Rational (and moral) actions, in this view, are those which are consistent with these human ends.[18] In short, Thomas's theory of natural moral obligation is constructed from his teleology of proper human inclinations. The primary precepts of the natural law are according to an order of primary natural inclinations (*ST* I–II,94,2): the tendency toward self-preservation, which humans share with every natural substance; the inclination to beget and educate offspring, which we share with all animals; and the inclination to apply reason, which is specific to humans and would include tendencies to know the truth about God, to live in society, to shun ignorance, etc. (McCormick's own description of basic human inclinations, listed in Section 2 above, corresponds in its essentials with Thomas's.) Secondary, and more specific, precepts of the natural law are rationally derived from these primary precepts. Thomas notes that some secondary precepts are not unconditional and absolute moral obligations, as their application might be "injurious" and therefore "unreasonable" in some circumstances.[19] Other precepts are, however, absolute and unconditional. For example, as has already been noted, the Thomistic tradition has consistently held that some sexual acts such as masturbation and contraceptive sterilization are always wrong in and of themselves. They are wrong because they are "unnatural" in their lack of orientation toward their proper natural end (procreation and education of children) with respect to their "form" (interior intentionality) or their "matter" (external object – i.e., insemination).[20]

One purpose of this explication of Thomas's teleology and its derived absolute moral prohibitions is to call attention to *why* McCormick insists upon re-describing these intrinsically "unnatural" (and "morally evil") actions as "premoral" evils, since this move has been the basis of some traditionalists' criticism that McCormick wants to throw all evils onto the same scale for 'weighing' in consequentialist fashion. John Connery observes, with particular reference to the sexual evils of masturbation and sterilization, that the Church has "always assumed that these acts are wrong *because* they are against the good of marriage . . . [whereas McCormick implies] that these acts are wrong *when* they are against the good of marriage" ([15], p. 495). While Connery's aim is to critique proportionalism for its "ambiguity" in exceptionmaking, his observation is right on target. For while McCormick, like Thomas, has no intention of relativizing the basic goods to which we are all naturally inclined, he also insists that we must not ignore all we have learned from the empirical and social sciences over the past seven centuries in our determination of *whether* a particular sexual act is "unnatural" in the sense of being against the good of marriage. Certainly any reasonable person who shared Thomas's thirteenth-century understanding of biology, metaphysics, the limitations of medical science, etc., would probably concur that masturbation always violates the natural *telos* of sexuality. But what about the reasonable person of the late twentieth century? Is it against the good of marriage, for example, for a husband to produce a sperm sample for infertility testing and treatment, or even for artificial insemination of his wife?[21] Or, is the good of marriage violated when a woman who has as many children as she can feed and educate already (and whose life would be endangered by another pregnancy) chooses contraception or sterilization rather than abstaining from sexual intimacy with her husband?[22] In McCormick's view, examples such as these illustrate (at the level of common sense) the unreasonableness of maintaining a purely 'physicalist' understanding of sexuality and its relation to its end. Thomas's teleological understanding of sexuality was essentially "read off of" observations of sexual purposiveness in all animals. But McCormick is arguing that we must certainly add to this our modern, expanded knowledge (of, e.g., medical possibility) in rationally assessing the directedness (or lack thereof) of sexual actions to their proper end.

In a similar vein, Peter Knauer has argued that in order for an action to be "proportionate" to its proper end it must not be a "counter-productive" (contradictory) means to that end "in the long run and in general." McCormick, in a generally favorable commentary on Knauer's proposal, suggests tentatively that the epistemological question of what is "counterproductive" is probably answered in different ways depending on the issue at stake ([42], p. 16f.). First, common experience gives us sound evidence that some actions are counterproductive (e.g., "We know that permanent marriage offers unsurpassable opportunities for human fulfillment, hence that actions that undermine its stability and permanence [adultery] are counterproductive"). Second, some actions provoke in us a very strong "sense" (intuition, or sense of profanation) that they are counterproductive; our revulsion makes us "grateful that we have not as yet had the experience." And third, there are some actions or procedures whose possible counterproductivity we know little about, so that we must "proceed to normative statements gradually by trial and error." (Our moral statements about recombinant DNA research are cited as belonging in this category.) Interestingly, McCormick concludes with a lament that, "[p]erhaps the mechanizing and quantifying of moral judgements that occurred during several centuries of high casuistry has led us to expect a type of certainty in some moral judgements that is beyond realistic expectation" ([42], p. 17). Be that as it may, McCormick himself must be somewhat confident of our epistemological ability to recognize the 'fit' between actions and their ends. For he is claiming, in essence, that his moral theory will allow exceptions to some of the Thomistic tradition's unexceptionable rules on the same end-oriented grounds which led Thomas to make them unexceptionable in the first place: namely, a teleology of human inclinations and of actions which *we can understand to be* properly directed toward those inclinational ends.

Utilitarianism: One teleological model of moral obligation which found classical expression in the nineteenth century is "Utilitarianism." Its principal founders, Jeremy Bentham (1748–1832) and John Stuart Mill (1806–1873), understood the morally proper *telos* of human actions to be "net social good." In this view, obligatory acts are those demanded by the principle of utility, i.e., those which will produce the greatest possible balance of (non-moral) good over evil in the world. Bentham and Mill identified the good hedonistically – that is, in terms of happiness or pleasure (both physical and psychological). Therefore, utility was for them a matter of maximizing pleasure and minimizing pain for all persons concerned. Further, "net social good" meant for both of them that maximizing the greatest good for the greatest number might require *not* maximizing the good – or even producing its opposite – for a minority.[24]

Later utilitarians have offered reformulations of classical utilitarianism which redefine either the nature of the good to be maximized or the form of the moral obligation involved. Non-hedonistic or "ideal" utilitarians (like

G.E. Moore) have emphasized such values as knowledge, beauty, aesthetic experience and personal affections, for example, as constitutive of the human 'good.' More recently, some utilitarians have promoted a "preferential" form of the theory in which the good to be maximized is the collection of the 'goods' of all involved individuals as determined (or "preferred") by the individuals themselves.

As for the nature of utilitarian moral obligation, the classical theory has given birth to both "act" and "rule" forms. Act-utilitarians hold that one should appeal directly to the principle of utility in every situation of choice. Thus one must always ask, "Will *this action* produce the greatest net social good of all available alternatives?" The role of rules in determining moral obligation is a very limited one for the act-utilitarian; rules merely provide a "summary" of accumulated wisdom about those actions in the past which have tended to maximize utility, and thus are useful only as rules of thumb and not in determining rightness/wrongness of particular acts. The rule-utilitarian, on the other hand, judges particular acts to be right or wrong on the basis of their conformity to or violation of valid rules of conduct; the validity of those rules of conduct is in turn determined by their tendency to promote utility if consistently followed. So, the rule-utilitarian, in contrast to the act-utilitarian, accepts (utility-validated) rules of conduct as the *criteria* of right and wrong action.

It should be noted that some philosophers consider act- and rule-utilitarianism to be extensionally equivalent (see, e.g., [59]). Their argument centers upon the logic of exception-making. For, the rule-utilitarian inevitably will face conflicts between valid rules of conduct; when he does, he will need a "second-order" moral rule to determine which obligation is heavier, and that second-order rule can be none other than the principle of utility itself. Thus, the argument goes, at least in conflict situations the rule-utilitarian must allow for exceptions to his rules which appeal directly to utility. Rule-utilitarians themselves often counter this argument by pointing to cases (e.g., acts of cheating or bribery) which would be judged wrong on rule-utilitarian grounds but which would be wrong for the act-utilitarian only if they were made public (with the resultant disutility of eroding public trust, etc.). And, in the rule-utilitarian's view, his understanding of norms of practice reflects more closely the actual moral judgements of reasonable people than that of the act-utilitarian. So, debate about the incompatibility or extensional equivalence of these two forms of utilitarianism has not issued in any consensus.

To summarize this overview of types of utilitarian theory, then, we might say that utilitarianism holds as the single ultimate standard of right, wrong, and obligation the principle of utility, which states that the ultimate goal of our actions (or rules of conduct) should be the greatest possible balance of non-moral good over evil in the world ([22], p. 34).

Consequentialism: The term "consequentialism" was coined by G.E.M.

Anscombe in 1958 to refer to the theories of "every single English academic moral philosopher since Sidgwick" ([1], p. 10). This "shallow philosophy" proposes, on Anscombe's reading, that right actions are those which in the actor's judgement will produce the best total consequences; the consequentialist's *standards* for judging consequences are invariably "the standards current in his society or circle." Thus he is condemned to be conventional, and "the chance that a whole range of conventional standards will be decent is small." Moreover, the consequentialist perverts the very notion of a moral 'ought,' which in our history is derived from the *law* conception of ethics introduced in the Hebrew-Christian tradition, by denying what is "characteristic" of that tradition – namely, that some actions are forbidden "whatever *consequences* threaten." In effect, Anscombe is labelling as consequentialist any moral theory which does not designate certain identifiable *kinds of action* as *always* right or wrong without any regard to consequences whatever. So her wide net includes even the rule-deontological Oxford Intuitionists (W.D. Ross et al.), who

... of course distinguish between 'consequences' and 'intrinsic values' and so produce a misleading appearance of not being 'consequentialists.' But they do not hold – and Ross explicitly denies – that the gravity of. e.g., procuring the condemnation of the innocent is such that it cannot be outweighed by, e.g., national interest. Hence their distinction is of no importance ([1], p. 9, n. 1).

Anscombe distinguishes between "old-fashioned Utilitarianism" and "consequentialism" by pointing out that the latter denies any moral distinction between one's responsibility for *intended* evil consequences and for merely *foreseen* consequences, while the former theory preserved that distinction. (Bentham, for instance, distinguished between evils "directly" intended and those only "obliquely" intended.) Of the two theories, then, consequentialism represents for Anscombe the less sophisticated or morally sensitive approach to maximizing good outcomes.

Much of the subsequent literature, however, has either treated "consequentialism" as more-or-less synonymous with "utilitarianism" (in its "greatest good for the greatest number" sense) or has referred to the latter as a "type" of the former without suggesting what any other "types" of consequentialism might look like.[25] McCormick at one point (in 1970) identified Joseph Fletcher's act-utilitarianism as "Fletcherian consequentialism," and, while rejecting that theory, went on to speculate that perhaps "there is a rendering of consequentialism, as yet not systematically developed, with which many of us could feel at home" ([39], p. 295, n. 14). Of course, McCormick has never admitted to feeling "at home" with anything like "utilitarianism"; quite the contrary! And it is interesting that, as his own moral theory has become more and more refined over time, McCormick's willingness to associate the term "consequentialist" with himself has steadily diminished (as a chronological reading of his "Notes on Moral Theology" series will attest). In the early 1970's, for example, he pointed approvingly to examples of "consequentialist analysis" or "consequentialist methodology"; more recently, however, he is critical of the "jargon" of "consequentialist" and even "proportionalist" when applied to revisionist moral theologians (including himself). Perhaps he now believes he is less consequentialist than he once was; or perhaps he has despaired of ever separating the term itself from the negative conceptual baggage heaped upon it by Anscombe and others; or perhaps both are true. In any case, it is the issue of how much weight consequences *are* given in McCormick's teleology to which we now turn.

To begin with, some of McCormick's early examples of proportionate reasoning display a clearly consequentialist bent. In his 1973 Pere Marquette Lecture, a restudy of the principle of double effect published as *Ambiguity in Moral Choice* [32], he argued that "judicial murder" (in order to prevent mob violence) and counter-population bombing (in order to end a war sooner) are both disproportionate because of their "long-term effects." Commenting upon the Catholic Church's traditionally absolute principle of discrimination (noncombatant immunity) he suggested that,

> ... it is precisely because of foreseen consequences that such a principle is a practical absolute. In this perspective its meaning would be: even though certain short-term advantages might be gained by taking innocent life in wartime, ultimately and in the long run, the harm would far outweigh the good ... Taking innocent human life as a means removes restraints and unleashes destructive powers which both now and in the long run will brutalize sensitivities and take many more lives than we would now save by such action. We cannot prove this type of assertion with a syllogistic click, but it is a good human bet given our knowledge of ourselves and our history – at least good enough to generate a practically exceptionless imperative, the type of moral rule Donald Evans refers to as 'virtually exceptionless' ([32], p. 42).

Similarly, McCormick was "strongly inclined" in another 1973 article to consider the rule against voluntary, active euthanasia of the terminally ill as "absolute" [33]. After reviewing some of the possible effects of altering that rule (e.g., capricious application, altering the traditional physician-patient relationship, eroding health professionals' attitudes of mercy, etc.), he concluded that we should recognize its "prudential validity" by analogy to positive laws established on the presumption of a common and universal danger: "Its sense is that even if the action in question does not threaten the individual personally, there remains the further presumption that to allow individuals to make that decision for themselves will pose a threat for the common good."[26]

These examples of proportionality are on any account the kind of reasoning one might expect from some utilitarians, specifically rule-utilitarians. However, McCormick's more recent methodological moves have included attempts to clarify and emphasize the non-utilitarian character of his method. His more current analysis of, e.g., judicial murder, Mrs. Bergmeier's adultery, and counter-population bombing (as presented in Section 2, above) represent this transition. Gone is the simple "long-term effects" justification of, say, the rule of non-combatant immunity; it has been replaced by a criterion of intrinsic "necessity" of means, particularly in terms of the disproportion of turning against "associated basic goods" in one's choices.

We should note here, though, that these alterations in McCormick's ethical method have failed to satisfy many of those critics who consider his "proportionalism" thoroughly consequentialist in stripe. Among the most prominent of those critics is John Finnis (see, e.g., [21]). Finnis insists that McCormick's new "key concept" – i.e., that denial of one basic value undermines the other basic value being sought (through the association of basic goods) – is a notion "entirely dependent for its intelligibility on the (speculatively supposed) *long run*" ([21], p. 101). In other words, Finnis reads McCormick as meaning that any denial of the sought value will come only as a *result* or *consequence* of one's immediate denial of an associated basic value; it becomes, then, just another (albeit weighty) evil result to be weighed in a calculus of consequences.

Further, citing the above examples of judicial murder and bombing, Finnis avers that McCormick's linkage between denial of liberty (through judicial or military "extortion") and denial of the good of life itself is the product of "an altogether mysterious process of speculative 'association of good'" ([21], p. 103). That process – be it a matter of instinct, intuition, or whatever – does not provide for us clear, rational grounds for McCormick's conclusions, but only "diverting rationalizations" for conclusions he has reached on other, clearly consequential grounds. Indeed, as Finnis sees it,

Once a moralist accepts proportionalist method, even as one methodological principle amonst [sic] others, he can produce arguments in favour of any solution which he already favours. All such arguments will be illegitimate, i.e., mere rationalizations ([21], p. 95).

Finally, Finnis complains that McCormick's emphases upon long-term evil effects and upon the denial of associated basic goods have meant that the basic value immediately at stake (e.g., the lives of innocents directly killed in terror-bombing) "disappears from – or never gets into – the moral focus." Or, more strongly, the identification of actual evil and wrong even in "plain murder" is "implausible and misdirected" in McCormick's analysis ([21], p. 104).

This complaint reflects Finnis's most fundamental critique of any and all forms of 'proportionalism' (which includes, in his view, "utilitarianism" and "consequentialism") – namely, that they are not only "impracticable" but also "senseless" in that they propose to compare and weigh basic goods which are in fact "incommensurable" ([21], p. 109). These incommensurable goods include life, knowledge, play, aesthetic experience, sociability (friendship), practical reasonableness and religion. They are each *equally fundamental* aspects of human well-being; thus, to deny any of them directly for the sake of the others is actually to deny them all ([20], pp. 85–95, 118–25). And to deny any (all) of them based upon a mere *prediction* of *probable* value-affirming *consequences* is unreasonable – a further violation of the basic good of "practical reasonableness." Of course, rarely can we actively *pursue* all of the basic goods in any given choice, either. Some will almost inevitably be indirectly "damaged" in our promotion of others. Finnis's point, though (one he shares with, e.g., Germain Grisez), is that we can still "respect" those basic goods we are not immediately promoting, but we violate all of them whenever we *directly* and *intentionally* choose to act against any one of them:

> To choose an act which in itself simply (or primarily) damages a basic good is thereby to engage oneself willy-nilly (but directly) in an act of opposition to an incommensurable value (an aspect of human personality) which one treats as if it were an object of measurable worth that could be outweighed by commensurable objects of greater (or cumulatively greater) worth. To do this will often accord with our feelings, our generosity, our sympathy, and with our commitments and projects in the forms in which we undertook them. But it can never be justified in reason . . . Reason requires that every basic value be at least respected in each and every action ([20], p. 120).

McCormick's general response to this last criticism is outlined in Section 2, above. He agrees that any direct and intentional "turning against" a basic good constitutes moral evil. But he also insists that some deliberate choices against a basic good – i.e., where its denial is not "approved of" in the agent's will, where its sacrifice clearly is causally necessary to prevent further, greater sacrifice of basic goods, and where the choice does not involve denial of other "associated goods" – do not constitute "turning against" that good at all. Finnis, however, sees in this explanation an unreasonable exercise of speculative prediction (about values to be preserved as a *consequence* of one's action) and a "mysterious" appeal to the notion of associated basic goods. In his view, we step beyond the limits of "practical reasonableness" when we try to justify our choices by looking *beyond* the basic goods we promote, "respect" or deny in our acts themselves.

Notwithstanding his differences with Finnis about what it means to "turn against" a basic good, and about whether the denial of an associated basic good (in some actions against a basic good) is "intrinsic" to that choice or merely a "consequence" of it, McCormick would deny vigorously Finnis's essential identification of "proportionalism" with "consequentialism" and "utilitarianism." First of all, certain features of McCormick's teleology distinguish it from either act- or rule-utilitarian approaches. We have seen, for example, that his use of the term "premoral evil" does not mean that actions which embody these disvalues are morally neutral in themselves. Unless a higher, conflicting value is at stake, a premoral evil is *morally* to be avoided because it is something already recognized to be lacking in orientation toward the *telos* of human flourishing. In other words, we don't have to *first* assess the consequences of a particular action (or rule of practice) in order to determine its prima facie evil (or good) qualities; we know these qualities "prediscursively." And thus it is simply moral common sense (personal and collective) which usually tells us what is of value (i.e., "an intrinsic good to man") and what constitutes, *ceteris paribus*, moral obligation in everyday life.

McCormick has concentrated so much on choice-making in moral *conflicts* – that is, situations in which protection of one value will invariably involve sacrifice of another – that these "intrinsic" right-making (or wrong-making) features of actions involving premoral values (or disvalues) are often overlooked or misunderstood by his readers. But those who claim to understand what he is saying about premoral values and moral obligation tend to describe his theory as something other than truly consequentialist. Peter Singer, for example, who describes himself as a consequentialist, is methodologically unsatisfied with the importance McCormick gives to intrinsic values of actions apart from consequence-calculation:

> I find McCormick's general position, though defensible, unpersuasive because I find it hard to find any intrinsic disvalue in, say, promise-breaking, apart from the bad effect that breaking a promise may have on those who expected it to be kept, and on promising itself ([57], p. 44).

In Singer's estimation, the practical difference between a teleological theory that includes such intrinsic values and a deontological ethic of prima facie duties "dwindles to nothing." Speaking as a consequentialist, then, Singer does not consider McCormick an ally.[27]

A second point of distinction between McCormick's theory and consequentialist theories has to do with the nature of the *telos* in each. At the center of utilitarian theories is a quantitative notion of "the greatest good for the greatest number" or "net social good" as the *telos* of actions or rules of practice. The good in question is defined in temporal, physical or psycho-social terms; and it is assumed to be *limited* good, since 'utility' is essentially a principle of distribution of it. McCormick's theory, on the other hand, shares with other Thomistic theories a notion of ultimate good (*summum bonum*) that is non-temporal, unlimited, and unquantifiable. This transcendent *telos* is the standard of all lesser goods, thus restricting their quantifiability as well. Therefore, McCormick's theory allows for conceptions of human dignity and human rights that are not determined by or overridable for consequentialist advantage. This is illustrated in his criterion of "necessity": abortion, for example, is justifiable only when the fetus (and mother) would die anyway without it and the value of the mother's life can be concretely preserved with it. The value of the fetus's life cannot morally be "weighed" against other values (e.g., the mother's convenience or family finances). And, as Lisa Cahill has cogently observed, "[a] relevant premise in calculations of proportion having to do with human rights or human life is that human dignity does not increase or decrease in quantity by the addition or subtraction of the individuals in whom it inheres" ([7], p. 616, n. 4; see also [8]). In short, calculations of the community's "net social good" cannot, in McCormick's theory, override or outweigh the value of individual human dignity, which is oriented toward the transcendent *telos* of humanity.

Another way of looking at this issue is in terms of the moral principles of beneficence and justice. Simply put, utilitarian theories tend to give priority to beneficence over justice (or at least to define the latter in terms of ultimate maximization of the former). Indeed, the utilitarian determines the justice of an action or rule of practice according to its overall promotion of net benefit; individual rights are recognized as valid only insofar as their observance can be seen to be conducive to overall benefit for the community. But this cannot be said of McCormick's moral theory. His teleology presupposes a conception of human rights as justifiable claims grounded in intrinsic dignity-values, which cannot be outweighed by any broader community-benefit assessment.[28] Rather, recognition of these values (and rights) is a precondition of the possibility of the community's orientation toward its genuine *telos* ([7], pp. 624–27). In other words, justice-claims are not incompatible with or subservient to benefit-maximization in this view; they are instead foundational for its realization and provide a framework for its interpretation. This does not mean that all personal rights (e.g., the fetus's right to life) are untouchable in situations of value-conflict. But it does mean that persons are protected in ways (and for reasons) that utilitarian theorists would not admit.

A good example of the centrality of justice-claims in McCormick's thought is his justification of (some) non-therapeutic research involving children. He does *not* argue that minimal-risk research is justified because the risks to the child-subject are outweighed by the potential benefits to other children; nor does he argue that a rule allowing use of children in such research would redound to overall net social good in the long run. Rather, he appeals to justice-claims in his assumption of what the child *ought* to want and thus *would* want if competent to consent, and also in recognizing limits to what can be expected of the child. First, the child would assumedly consent to beneficial research with "no discernible risk or undue discomfort" if he could, because that would be a reasonable acceptance of his "fair share" of the burden of medical progress which allows all children to prosper. The child's own "flourishing" includes, in McCormick's view, some minimal involvement in the flourishing of his peers. Second, the child's innate human dignity – and thus his human rights – must not be violated by exposing him to more-than-minimal risk; for to do so would be to "use" the child for the benefit of others, and that would be a quantification and trading-off of a non-quantifiable value. In sum, notions of social justice and human rights provide, in this example, a clear and restrictive framework which must be recognized prior to any assessment of beneficial consequences to the community.

A third non-consequentialist feature of McCormick's teleology, following from the two just mentioned, is his treatment of exceptionless moral norms.

As we have seen, he posits one clear moral absolute: one must never deliberately induce another to do that which either party believes to be moral evil. The rationale for this norm is teleological (in that it recognizes a person's moral integrity as his highest good in life, orienting him toward his *summum bonum*) but not consequentialist, since it cannot be overridden by any appeal to immediate or long-term consequences. It also follows from the same rationale that it is absolutely wrong to do moral evil oneself – one must never be unjust, unfaithful, untruthful, etc. Because the determination of what actions *are* morally evil often involves a "weighing of some sort" of premoral evils in value-conflicts, and because "middle axioms" of moral obligation are derived from these determinations, it is apparent that McCormick's method does bear practical "structural similarities" with rule-utilitarianism, as Childress suggests. But substantive dissimilarities are also apparent, inasmuch as McCormick's theory of value emphasizes human dignity-values which are not temporal goods as such and which cannot be overridden by considerations of utility. So, while specific "virtually exceptionless" rules determined by proportionate reason might indeed coincide with those determined on rule-utilitarian grounds (or, for that matter, on rule-deontological grounds), the particular values to be weighed in that determination – and the hierarchy within which they are considered – may be quite different from those emphasized in utilitarian teleology.

Given these considerations, it would seem reasonable to accept McCormick's insistence that his ethical method represents neither pure consequentialism nor pure deontology but rather, as he puts it, a "moderate teleology" – or "mixed consequentialism," as Charles Curran describes it.[29] But we should also note, in closing, that the hierarchical understanding of values which grounds "proportionate reason" is also the source of its greatest complexity and unclarity as an ethical theory. For, McCormick and other "proportionalists" are attempting to 'update' the notion of the *ordo bonorum* and to clarify for modern understanding the relations of its constituent goods. But the problem this attempt poses for McCormick's ethical method is, in the words of one of his most sympathetic critics, that ". . . in the absence of a classical or medieval metaphysics and anthropology, it is no mean task to discern and agree upon the precise relations of values in the hierarchy upon which the theory depends" ([7], p. 617). McCormick frequently implies that particular conclusions reached theoretically through proportionate reasoning are more immediately available through good moral common sense. This may well be so; but it does not solve the theoretician's problem of finding clear and compelling conceptual validations for those conclusions. Clarity and simplicity are certainly cardinal virtues for a moral theory.

One area of value-relation within the *ordo bonorum* which is in urgent need of further explication is the "association of basic goods." We have noted McCormick's assertion that, in practice, recognition of these associated goods will place limitations upon any simple consequentialist calculus in moral conflict situations. None of the associated basic goods may be suppressed deliberately except where it is *necessary* – i.e., "the only way possible, essentially and deterministically" – for the achievement of other basic goods in the situation of choice ([37], p. 261). But why exactly do these particular basic values (as listed in Section 2, above) constitute the association? And, further, are they all *equally* basic? Cahill has pointed out that while they are all "fundamental in some sense," they don't seem to be "equally and absolutely" so in McCormick's discussion of them ([7], p. 623). This leaves open the possibility of a hierarchy of associated basic goods within the broader *ordo bonorum*. Given the importance (and weight) of this association in McCormick's moral theory, further clarification and defense of it would be most welcome. Certainly he needs to explain to Finnis – and the rest of us – why his appeals to it are not indeed "mysterious" and "speculative."

The moral theory advanced by contemporary "proportionalists" like McCormick is, in many respects, of a piece with the Thomistic tradition within which it has been nurtured. It is also very different, in other respects, from the manualist tradition and much of contemporary neo-Thomism. Perhaps the most fundamental difference lies in the notion of practical agential responsibility. For, while the many casuistical 'absolutes' of the manualists painted a rather strict and demanding picture of moral goodness, they also provided a sort of spiritual 'safety' in their ostensive objective certainty. In contrast, revisionist moral theologians have challenged the very foundations of that agent-security with their frank admissions of "ambiguity in moral choice." To the Protestant observer (such as the present writer) this shift appears to imply also a new recognition of the finitude and sinfulness that surround moral responsibility, with a resultant awareness of the possibility of truly "tragic" choices and a relative de-emphasis on the tradition's sometimes-excessive concern for moral self-justification – all of which have been typically "Protestant" concerns. Viewed in this light, McCormick and other revisionist theorists might be seen to be cultivating common ground for productive self-analysis (and mutual criticism) of both traditions.

Protestantism does not, of course, have any single, clearly defined 'tradition' of moral theology to parallel the Catholic natural law tradition. One might even say that "revisionist moral theology" would be the descriptive *norm* of Protestantism rather than the exception! And the next three chapters will indeed offer illustration of the striking diversity of Protestant perspectives on moral being and doing.

NOTES

[1] Thomas Aquinas held that "natural law" – the moral law of the universe – is a subset of the "eternal law" which exists in the mind of God. "Divine law" is another part of the eternal law,

ORDERED VALUES AND PROPORTIONATE REASONS 49

given by God to humanity through direct revelation. And "human law" is that collection of norms which human beings legislate for their own behavior in civil community.

[2] In the Thomistic framework, for example, masturbation constituted a greater sin against the *natural* law than did rape, since the latter involved a closer approximation of the proper "natural" function of the sexual organs. (Of course, rape constituted a most heinous offense against *human* law.)

[3] Pope Paul VI's condemnation of artificial contraception in *Humanae Vitae* (1968) – alluded to above in Chapter 1 – follows from his reasoning about the objective "nature" of marriage and sexuality which, in my view, certainly represents the "Greek" influence in Thomistic natural law.

[4] See, e.g., [38], pp. 345ff., 358f., 395f.; and [48].

[5] Reported in the *Journal of the American Medical Association* 227 (1974), 728.

[6] Pius XII, *Acta Apostolicae Sedis*, 49 (1957) 1031–32, cited in [38], 345f.; see also [34], p. 77, and [40], p. 321.

[7] John D. Arras believes McCormick has confused his relational potential standard with a best-interests-of-the-child standard, in part because McCormick once referred to the capacity for human relationships as a "summary" of the hardship/benefit criterion (Cf. [53], p. 316). Thus Arras thinks that McCormick does have a working standard for cases in which a child faces relationship-obscuring pain or future suffering, but not for cases in which the child's "lack of capacity for personal relations is due to a lack of awareness unaccompanied by pain" ([2], pp. 25–33). What Arras fails to see is that McCormick has also advanced a 'prospect of benefit' standard, based also upon relational potential, which *does* apply in cases of infants whose existence is free of both pain and relational prospect. Indeed, McCormick notes at one point that if treatment of a defective neonate would result in a life "without meaningful relationships," then that treatment "is not *medically* indicated" ([43], p. 22).

[8] [53], p. 317. In an earlier article, co-authored with Robert Veatch ("The Preservation of Life and Self-Determination," [38], pp. 371–79), McCormick argues for two principles to be applied in medical decision-making for incompetents: the principle of patient benefit and the principle of "familial self-determination." The authors go on to state that when the familial judgement about the incompetent person's best interests "so exceeds the limits of reason" that it cannot be tolerated by society, then often "a public official such as a judge" may have to be called upon to protect the patient's best interests.

[9] McCormick follows several contemporary Continental moral theologians in elucidating this distinction. Joseph Fuchs, S.J. uses the term "premoral evil"; Bruno Schuller, S.J., "nonmoral evil"; and Louis Janssens, "ontic evil" – all as essentially synonymous with the manualists' "physical evil."

[10] See [37], esp. pp. 254–65. Schüller's basic claim is that one must never intentionally (approvingly) cause another to sin (do moral evil). McCormick's addition (related in a personal conversation with this writer December 9, 1987) is that we should never intentionally cause another to do what we know he/she believes to be moral evil. Of course, this raises the issue of justifiable or forbidden violations of individual *conscience* – an issue McCormick should attend to more substantially, given its importance in this context.

[11] See, e.g., [38], 425f.; [32], pp. 7–51; [37], pp. 193–265; and [39], pp. 718–23.

[12] See [12], esp. pp. 12–21, for a discussion of various definitions of paternalism.

[13] Joel Feinberg has described the distinction between "weak" and "strong" paternalism. See [18], pp. 105–24, and [19], p. 33.

[14] It is interesting that much of what McCormick says about treatments which a conscious, competent patient ought to choose for himself appear in the context of his arguments about what treatments a third party ought to choose for an incompetent patient in specific cases. See, for example, his discussions of the Quinlan case in "The Moral Right to Privacy" and "The Quality of Life, the Sanctity of Life"; of the Saikewicz case in "The Case of Joseph Saikewicz" (with

Andre Hellegers); and of the Brother Fox case in "The Preservation of Life and Self-Determination" (with Robert Veatch) – all reprinted in [38]. This peripheral approach to the issue of patient autonomy – which is a *central* concern for so many contemporary philosophers and theologians – tends to underscore McCormick's commitment to an objective order of values which should guide *both* personal and third-party decision-making in much the same manner.

[15] See, for example, [10], [13], [14], [15], [23], [25], [50], [51], and [54].

[16] [7], p. 603. This article, along with Cahill's other reflections on McCormick's work, has also provided clear foundations for many of the points developed later in this section. I am, therefore, much indebted to Cahill, even if the notes that follow do not fully reflect that indebtedness.

[17] Ross, W.D.: 1939, *The Foundations of Ethics*, Clarendon, Oxford, p. 5, cited by Cahill in [7], p. 603.

[18] John Langan, S.J., has argued that Thomas's moral theory is not as teleological as it looks, because acting morally is not in itself a sufficient *cause* of perfect beatitude and because Thomas's various precepts of the natural law do not all appear (to Langan) to be deduced from our "natural tendencies." So Langan interprets these precepts as representing "a kind of deontological intuitionism" (see [29]). Lisa Cahill points out, though, that while supernatural beatitude is not caused by human acts in Thomas's view, natural, temporal fulfillment *is* so caused. Moreover, human acts resulting from grace-infused virtues do cause conformity to the supernatural end (see [7], p. 604, n. 8). There is indeed plenty of evidence in the Thomistic corpus for F.C. Copleston's assessment that the idea of the good is paramount in Thomas's ethical theory and that "human acts derive their moral quality from their relation to man's final end" (see [17], p. 206).

[19] For example, Thomas held that reason dictates a secondary precept that "goods entrusted to another should be restored to their owner." However, in some circumstances – e.g., if the goods are claimed for use in waging war against one's country – it would be reasonable *not* to restore them. McCormick would surely point to this as an example of "proportionate reasoning."

[20] Admittedly, this interpretation assumes a consistency in Thomas's linkage of moral obligation with natural teleology which Langan essentially rejects (see note 18, above) and denies Langan's suggestion that an independent theory of "deontological intuitionism" is at work in Thomas's secondary precepts.

[21] McCormick counts himself among those moral theologians who would not refer to self-stimulation in such circumstances as 'masturbation' at all, since that term generally has implied narcissistic intent.

[22] It must be admitted here that McCormick (along with a great many other modern moral theologians) differs with Thomas somewhat as to what the "good of marriage" itself involves. Thomas considered procreation to be the single legitimating purpose of sexual intercourse; marital enjoyment of sex was permissible as long as it was not the specific purpose of the sex act. Modern moral theologians describe the good of marriage in broader sociological and psychological terms, and many include the conjugal relational aspect of marital sex as a central feature of the good of marriage itself (and thus a proper *telos* of coitus).

[23] Knauer, P.: 1980, 'Fundamentalethik: Teleologische als Deontologische Normenbegrundung', *Theologie und Philosophie* 55, 321–60, cited by McCormick in 'Notes on Moral Theology: 1980' ([42], esp. pp. 12–17).

[24] Some defenders of utilitarianism, responding to the criticism that utility seems to make the good of some persons expendable, have countered that the overall, long-term good of everyone will probably be best served by consistently respecting certain minimal rights for every individual. Of course, if that particular cause-and-effect relation (between respecting rights and promoting general utility) should ever seem less convincing, then the (utilitarian) moral rationale for respecting those rights would be forfeit.

[25] Kurt Baier defines consequentialism as "the principle that consequences alone determine the rightness of an act, i.e., that the only right-making property of an act is its optimificity."

This involves both a denial of the intrinsic rightness of any non-optimific act and, more particularly, a denial of absolutism (i.e., the claim that certain types of acts are wrong whatever the consequences). In Baier's view, the rule-utilitarian does justify some non-optimific acts but would deny absolutism; the act-utilitarian is fully "consequentialist" in denying both intrinsicism and absolutism [3]. On the other hand, R.M. Hare defines utilitarianism as "a type of *consequentialism*, holding that the morality of actions is to be judged by their consequences" [26].

[26] [33], p. 319. It should be pointed out parenthetically that some rule-deontologists (e.g., Paul Ramsey, the subject of the next chapter) can justify some particular acts of mercy-killing but would also defend a rule against its practice on grounds very similar to McCormick's (though not within his methodology per se).

[27] Of course, one definitional question which arises at this point is, What counts as a *consequence*? Moral philosophy and theology do not offer an univocal answer. Is the "expression of solidarity" in one's action, or the intrinisic fidelity-value of promise-keeping, really an independent right-making quality of an action itself, or is it an *effect* or consequence of it? As we have seen, Anscombe (a deontologist of the 'absolutist' variety) denies any genuine distinction beween these "intrinsic" considerations and other, more material *effects*; both are, in her view, merely factors in a consequentialist calculus. On the other hand, though, Singer (along with many others) clearly accepts the distinction. And he applies it as evidence that McCormick's moral theory cannot be considered a "straightforward consequentialism." I would join Singer and McCormick in assuming that the intrinsic disvalue of an action does not have to be a consequence or effect of it (at least not in the sense in which we normally use those terms). For, Anscombe seems committed to the position that any argument which would claim that an action can be *intrinsically* wrong without being *absolutely* wrong must be a consequentialist argument; and such a position seems to offer only dogmatic categorization and not any practical pursuasiveness.

[28] Human rights are not always *absolute* claims of individuals in McCormick's view, as we saw in his arguments about the right of patient self-determination (Section 3). But even in that case, the right in question is not morally overridable for the broader benefit of others; it may be interfered with only when it is being abused (that is, when it is exercised in such a way as to threaten the objective 'best interests' of the person in question).

[29] See [39], esp. p. 651f. John Langan has even suggested that McCormick is a "crypto-deontologist", since the latter's insistence on the protection of "associated basic goods" has led him to posit virtually exceptionless rules that have been identified by others on deontological grounds [30].

REFERENCES

1. Anscombe, G.E.M.: 1958, 'Modern Moral Philosophy', *Philosophy* 33, 1–19.
2. Arras, J.D.: 1984, 'Toward an Ethic of Ambiguity', *Hastings Center Report* 14/2, 25–33.
3. Baier, K.: 1978, 'Ethics: Teleological Theories', in W.T. Reich (ed.), *Encyclopedia of Bioethics*, vol. 1, The Free Press, New York, pp. 417–21.
4. Blanchfield, D.: 1974, 'Methodology and McCormick', *American Ecclesiastical Review* 168/6, 372–89.
5. Broad, C.D.: 1930, *Five Types of Ethical Theory*, Routledge and Kegan Paul, London.
6. Cahill, L.S.: 1979, 'Within Shouting Distance: Paul Ramsey and Richard McCormick on Method', *Journal of Medicine and Philosophy* 4/4, 398–417.
7. Cahill, L.S.: 1981, 'Teleology, Utilitarianism, and Christian Ethics', *Theological Studies* 42, 601–29.
8. Cahill, L.S.: 1984, 'Contemporary Challenges to Exceptionless Moral Norms', in *Moral Theology Today: Certitudes and Doubts*, The Pope John Center, St. Louis, 121–35.

9. Cahill, L.S.: 1993, 'On Richard McCormick: Reason and Faith in Post-Vatican II Ethics', in A. Verhey and S.E. Lammers (eds.), *Theological Voices in Medical Ethics*, William B. Eerdmans, Grand Rapids, MI., pp. 78–105.
10. Carney, F.S.: 1978, 'On McCormick and Teleological Morality', *Journal of Religious Ethics* 6, 21–30.
11. Childress, J.F.: 1982 'Two by McCormick' (review of R.A. McCormick, *How Brave a New World?* and *Notes on Moral Theology, 1965–1980*), *Hastings Center Report* 12/3, 40–42.
12. Childress, J.F.: 1982, *Who Should Decide? Paternalism in Health Care*, Oxford University Press, New York.
13. Connery, J.R.: 1973, 'Morality of Consequences: A Critical Appraisal', *Theological Studies* 34, 396–414.
14. Connery, J.R.: 1981, 'Catholic Ethics: Has the Norm for Rule-Making Changed?' *Theological Studies* 42, 232–50.
15. Connery, J.R.: 1983, 'The Teleology of Proportionate Reason', *Theological Studies* 44, 489–96.
16. Connery, J.R.: 1984, 'The Basis for Certain Key Exceptionless Moral Norms', in *Moral Theology Today: Certitudes and Doubts*, The Pope John Center, St. Louis, MO., 182–92.
17. Copleston, F.C.: 1955, *Aquinas*, Penguin Books, New York.
18. Feinberg, J.: 1971, 'Legal Paternalism', *Canadian Journal of Philosophy* 1, 105–24.
19. Feinberg, J.: 1973, *Social Philosophy*, Prentice-Hall, Englewood Cliffs, NJ.
20. Finnis, J.: 1980, *Natural Law and Natural Rights*, Clarendon Press, Oxford.
21. Finnis, J.: 1983, *Fundamentals of Ethics*, Georgetown University Press, Washington, DC.
22. Frankena, W.: 1973, *Ethics*, 2nd ed., Prentice-Hall, Englewood Cliffs, NJ.
23. Frankena, W.: 1978, 'McCormick and the Traditional Distinction', in R.A. McCormick and P. Ramsey (eds.), *Doing Evil to Achieve Good*, Loyola University Press, Chicago, pp. 145–64.
24. Fuchs, J.: 1971, 'The Absoluteness of Moral Terms', *Gregorianum* 52, 415–58.
25. Grisez, G.: 1978, 'Against Consequentialism', *American Journal of Jurisprudence* 23, 21–72.
26. Hare, R.M.: 1978, 'Ethics: Utilitarianism', in W.T. Reich (ed.), *Encyclopedia of Bioethics*, vol 1, The Free Press, New York, pp. 424–29.
27. Janssens, L.: 1972, 'Ontic Evil and Moral Evil', *Louvain Studies* 4, 115–56.
28. Kelly, G.: 1957, *Medico-Moral Problems*, Catholic Hospital Association of the U.S. and Canada, St. Louis.
29. Langan, J.: 1977, 'Beatitude and Moral Law in St. Thomas', *Journal of Religious Ethics* 5/2, 183–95.
30. Langan, J.: 1979, 'Direct and Indirect – Some Recent Exchanges Between Paul Ramsey and Richard McCormick', *Religious Studies Review* 5, 95–101.
31. McCormick, R.A.: 1970, 'Christian Morals', *America* 122, 5.
32. McCormick, R.A.: 1973, *Ambiguity in Moral Choice*, Marquette University Theology Department, Milwaukee; reprinted in R.A. McCormick and P. Ramsey (eds.): 1978, *Doing Evil to Achieve Good: Moral Choice in Conflict Situations*, Loyola University Press, Chicago, pp. 7–53 (page references are to the latter volume).
33. McCormick, R.A.: 1973, 'The New Medicine and Morality', *Theology Digest* 21, 308–21.
34. McCormick, R.A.: 1975, 'A Proposal for "Quality of Life" Criteria for Sustaining Life', *Hospital Progress* 56/9, 76–79.
35. McCormick, R.A.: 1976, 'Experimental Subjects: Who Should They Be?' *Journal of the American Medical Association* 235, 2197.
36. McCormick, R.A.: 1976, 'Experimentation in Children: Sharing in Sociality', *Hastings Center Report* 6/6, 41–46.

37. McCormick, R.A.: 1978, 'A Commentary on the Commentaries', in R.A. McCormick and P. Ramsey (eds.), *Doing Evil to Achieve Good*, Loyola University Press, Chicago, pp. 193–267.
38. McCormick, R.A.: 1981, *How Brave a New World? Dilemmas in Bioethics*, Doubleday and Company, New York.
39. McCormick, R.A.: 1981, *Notes on Moral Theology, 1965–1980*, University Press of America, Lanham, MD.
40. McCormick, R.A.: 1882, 'Theology and Biomedical Ethics', *Eglise et Theologie* 13, 311–31. (Reprinted in *Logos* 3 [1983], 25–45.)
41. McCormick, R.A.: 1984, *Health and Medicine in the Catholic Tradition*, Crossroad, New York.
42. McCormick, R.A.: 1984, *Notes on Moral Theology, 1981–1984*, University Press of America, Lanham, MD.
43. McCormick, R.A.: 1986, 'The Best Interests of the Baby', *Second Opinion* 2, 18–25.
44. McCormick, R.A.: 1989, *The Critical Calling: Reflections on Moral Dilemmas Since Vatican II*, Georgetown University Press, Washington, D.C.
45. McCormick, R.A.: 1989, 'Theology and Bioethics', *Hastings Center Report* 19/2, 5–10.
46. McCormick, R.A.: 1990, 'Clear and Convincing Evidence: The Case of Nancy Cruzan', *Midwest Medical Ethics* 6 (Fall), 10–12.
47. McCormick, R.A.: 1991, 'Physician-Assisted Suicide: Flight from Compassion', *The Christian Century* 108, 1132–34.
48. McCormick, R.A.: 1992, '"Moral Considerations" Ill Considered', *America* 166/9, 210–14.
49. McCormick, R.A. and Tribe, L.H.: 1982, 'Infant Doe: Where to Draw the Line', *Washington Post*, July 27, A15.
50. MacIntyre, A.: 1979, 'Theology, Ethics, and the Ethics of Medicine and Health Care: Comments on Papers by Novak, Mouw, Roach, Cahill, and Hartt', *Journal of Medicine and Philosophy* 4, 435–43.
51. May, W.E.: 1978, 'The Moral Meaning of Human Acts', *Homiletic and Pastoral Review* 79/1, 10–21.
52. O'Connell, T.E.: 1976, *Principles for a Catholic Morality*, Seabury Press, New York.
53. Paris, J.J. and McCormick, R.A.: 1983, 'Saving Defective Infants: Options for Life and Death', *America* 148/16, 313–17.
54. Quay, P.M.: 1975, 'Morality by Calculation of Values', *Theology Digest* 23, 347–64.
55. Ramsey, P.: 1976, 'The Enforcement of Morals: Nontherapeutic Research on Children', *Hastings Center Report* 6/4, 21–30.
56. Schuller, B.: 1978, 'The Double Effect in Catholic Thought: A Reevaluation', in R.A. McCormick and P. Ramsey (eds.), *Doing Evil to Achieve Good*, Loyola University Press, Chicago, pp. 00.
57. Singer, P.: 1980, 'Do Consequences Count? Rethinking the Doctrine of Double Effect', *Hastings Center Report* 10/1, 42–44.
58. Spohn, W.C.: 1987, 'Richard A. McCormick: Tradition in Transition', *Religious Studies Review* 13/1, 39–42.
59. Taylor, P.W.: 1975, *Principles of Ethics: An Introduction*, Dickenson Publishing Co., Belmont, CA.
60. Walter, J.J.: 1990, 'The Foundation and Formulation of Norms', in C. Curran (ed.), *Moral Theology: Challenges for the Future*, Paulist Press, Mahwah, NJ, pp. 125–54.

CHAPTER THREE

PAUL RAMSEY:
AGAPE, "COVENANT FIDELITY," AND MORAL RULES

One of the peripheral lessons of the previous chapter is that diversity reigns within unity in contemporary Roman Catholic moral theology. As the next three chapters will illustrate, diversity may well be said to have the upper hand in contemporary Protestant ethics. Richard McCormick, as we have seen, has been criticized by many of his fellow Catholic moralists for rejecting so many of the tradition's moral 'absolutes.' Paul Ramsey, the Protestant ethicist to be considered in this chapter, has been criticized by many of his peers for *accepting* too many moral absolutes and insisting upon their quasi-casuistical application.

The past half century has seen the rise of several much-publicized trends or 'movements' in Protestant ethics: Reinhold Niebuhr's 'Christian pragmatism'; the love-oriented 'situational' ethics of John A. T. Robinson and Joseph Fletcher; and Paul Lehmann's 'contextualist' ethics, to name but a few. Paul Ramsey has been an outspoken critic of all of them. He agrees with Robinson and Fletcher about the centrality of love in Christian ethics, and he accepts many of Niebuhr's practical and theological-anthropological claims. But his particular interpretations of love's concrete requirements, of how we come to know those requirements, and of the proper method of applying them in moral life, all join to form a unique and complex moral perspective. Moreover, Ramsey's written corpus covers a wide range of topical and methodological arguments, and his approaches to specific ethical issues have been so varied as to prompt charges of inconsistency on his part. It is also true, however, that particular themes reappear again and again in his arguments about widely disparate topics; so it may be more accurate to say that his moral theory incorporates dialectically-related elements rather than simply to label it as inconsistent.

In any event, the genuine complexity of Ramsey's thought poses an immediate problem for any expositor of it: Where does one find an appropriate 'point of entry' into it? The approach taken in the first section of this chapter will be to deal with his early works chronologically, in order to indicate certain shifts of emphasis in the development of Ramsey's thought. The second section will be devoted to the role of moral norms – personal and social – in his moral theory. And the latter three sections will examine medico-moral applications of that theory.

AGAPE, "COVENANT FIDELITY," AND MORAL RULES 55

1. AGAPE AND COVENANT-FIDELITY: THEMATIC DEVELOPMENT

Ramsey's first book, *Basic Christian Ethics* [23], remains his only broad and fairly systematic treatise in theological ethics. That work, described by its author as "an essay in the Christocentric ethics of the Reformation," begins with the premise that the central ethical notion in Christianity is "obedient love" ([23], pp. xi, xiv). The full meaning of love (*agape*) is disclosed to us in the life and teachings of Jesus – this is what Ramsey means by calling his ethics "Christocentric" – but the referent notion of obedient love itself is rooted in the faith experience of Israel. The Bible's "main theme," Ramsey tells us, is the "righteousness of God" – his judgement and covenant faithfulness toward human beings. Because God's righteous judgements and saving activity are one, the biblical understanding of his righteousness recognizes none of our common philosophical distinctions between "justice" and "love"; both notions are unified in God's steadfast covenant-fidelity toward humankind. Indeed, the qualities of "justice (*mishpat*), righteousness (*tsedeq*), and mercy (*chesed*), which are to be distinguished on first beginning to understand the Bible, prove on closer inspection not at all clearly distinguishable in their meaning and never separable in fact" ([23], p. 9). And it is the biblical conception of righteousness which provides "the meaning and measure of full human obligation" ([23], p. 3). Humankind's proper response to God's covenant righteousness is "grateful obedience or obedient gratitude." God's righteousness becomes the "plumb line" for measuring the rightness of all our human relationships, which means that our standard for treating each of our neighbors is "according to the measure of his real need" (since that is the measure of God's righteousness toward him) ([23], pp. 13–14). This means, further, that of the two central ethical questions – *What* is the good? and *Whose* good should be sought? – the latter is "the main, perhaps the only, concern of Christian ethics" ([23], p. 114). Ramsey assumes that knowing and seeking 'the good' is a matter of natural desire, whereas neighbor-love is the demand of covenant-obedience and defines what is 'right'. Thus, "Christian ethics is a deontological ethics, not an ethic of 'the good.'" Only *after* the Christian's "right relation" of directedness toward the neighbor and the neighbor's need is established does he seek "as a secondary though quite essential concern ... for his neighbor's sake to ascend whatever scale of values he might find reasonably creditable" ([23], p. 116). In other words (and in clear contrast with McCormick's perspective), Christian ethics cannot find proper expression in a moral theory that is primarily teleological, that seeks to define human 'goods' and then to deduce the most suitable means of attaining those goods. Perhaps Ramsey's sharpest statement of this belief is offered in a later work, *Deeds and Rules in Christian Ethics*:

Agape defines for the Christian what is right, righteous, obligatory to be done among men; it is not a Christian's definition of the good that better be done and much less is it a definition of the right way to the good . . .

Eschatology has at least this significance for Christian ethics in all ages: that reliance on producing *teloi*, or on doing good consequences, or on goal-seeking, has been decisively set aside . . . The Christian understanding of righteousness is therefore radically non-teleological. It means ready obedience to the *present* reign of God, the alignment of the human will with the Divine will that men should live together in covenant-love no matter what the morrow brings, even if it brings nothing ([29], p. 108f.).

In insisting upon the non-teleological nature of Christian ethics, Ramsey is rejecting not only consequentialist theories but also any moral theory centered around attainment of the self's *bonum* – even the *summum bonum* of fellowship with God (which Ramsey takes to be the teleological focus of Thomistic natural law theology). For, the "end-term" of *agape* is always the neighbor alone; his good is the only good sought. Any good for the self which might follow upon an act of Christian love follows "as quite unintended consequence."[1]

Given Ramsey's interpretation of "obedient love" as *the* norm of human conduct in *Basic Christian Ethics*, and given his insistence upon the radically non-teleological character of that norm, it remains to be asked, What form does this loving obedience take in practice? How do we know – and how do we best formulate – what love requires? Does it require the same response in every relevantly similar situation of choice, or does it require that each neighbor-relation be seen as making new and unique demands on us? Ramsey has offered somewhat varied answers to these questions over the years, marking a genuine development – some would say a profound conflict – in his understanding(s) of the role of rules in Christian moral life.

His original position, articulated in *Basic Christian Ethics*, is perhaps most boldly expressed in the chapter entitled (suggestively), "Christian Liberty: An Ethic Without Rules":

. . . Christians are bound by Jesus' attitude of sticking as close as possible to human need, no matter what the rules say, as the primary meaning of obligation . . . Strictly speaking, this is a new 'principle' for morality only in the sense that here all morality governed by principles, rules, customs, and laws goes to pieces and is given another sovereign test ([23], p. 57).

This statement is intended, in its context, as a rejection of *a priori*, strictly codified sets of moral rules; Ramsey is inveighing here primarily against the Catholic tradition of natural law morality. Rules, as general action-directions, are acceptable to him insofar as they are derived "backward" from what love sees as the needs of others. But any rules taught by 'nature' or by human intelligence alone – or even taught previously by love itself – "must always be held suspect enough for critical re-examination in the light of present neighbor-needs and the means available for meeting them" ([23], p. 81). In other words, love must occupy the "ground floor" in any genuinely Christian ethic. Later in the same volume, Ramsey admits that "Christian love in search of a social policy" may well need to incorporate the practical wisdom of natural law traditions and philosophical idealism; nevertheless, while *agape* "makes alliance or coalition with any available sources of insight or information about what should be done, it makes *concordat* with none of these" ([23], p. 344).

Moreover, as the moral legalism of natural law is dethroned by "obedient love," so also is the relative normlessness of theological intuitionism (or "intuitionism on stilts," as Ramsey calls it). Such intuitionism, of those in "so-called Barthian circles," is rejected for two reasons. First, it may derive ethical directives from the momentary "absolute demands" of God which contradict human conscience or natural reason, whereas true faith broadens and improves upon natural reason by addressing the problem of saving us from the *sinful* employment of whatever standards reason leads us to accept.[2] And, second, while theological intuitionism depends upon the "felt power or powerful feeling" of immediate divine command, Christian love (as directedness toward meeting the neighbor's need) offers a content-rich principle for discriminating among such intuitions according to their "specific quality" rather than simply their felt power ([23], p. 339). In summary, then, *Basic Christian Ethics* outlines an ethic of Christian love which is not "unruly" or feeling-dominant and which can "use" the insights of other theories of social ethics, but which "takes on the aspect of a quite indeterminate norm when compared with any and all forms of legalistic social ethics" ([23], p. 340). Such an ethic captures Luther's notion of "the freedom of a Christian": freedom *from* legalistic dogmas, freedom *for* the neighbor in his present need.[3]

Over the years, however, Ramsey's early "accent" on love's freedom has been refined, and perhaps replaced, by other accents. By 1960, the characteristic Lutheran theme of obedient "faith working through love" had become, for Ramsey, "faith effective through *in-principled* love." This latter phrase provided the title of an article which argues that a Christian ethic must be true to the Gospel while also including "principles, rules, law, habit, and a morphology of man." Love must work itself out concretely through principles, be they principles derived intrinsically from love itself or extrinsically from the perceived demands of natural justice [24].

In-principled love is elaborated further in *Christian Ethics and the Sit-In* (1961). In that volume, Ramsey approaches the traditional tensions between reason and revelation (or 'nature and grace,' or 'justice and love') through the theological categories of creation and redemption. He argues, following the language of Karl Barth, that God's covenant dealings with mankind presuppose God's ordering of human life in creation. And creation supplies its own sorts of norms for human life: natural justice; human and legal rights; civil law as an ordinance of creation; and social institutions. Such norms are the "external basis" which helps make possible the actualization of "the promise of the covenant." From the other direction, covenant (which Ramsey also equates with Barth's notion of "fellow humanity") is the "internal basis" of true justice, rights, or laws. Seen in this light, then, the requirements of steadfast covenant-love and of justice (or natural right) are "ultimately inseverable" ([25, pp. 22, 26).

As an example of this external/internal relation between justice and covenant-love, Ramsey offers his understanding of the human right of private property. Covenant-love means that we should live our lives *for* our fellow human beings, in full "fellow humanity." Life *for* others, however, must also be life *with* others; and natural justice, here in the form of property-rights, provides the requisite order of life *with* others. "Property, like all other rights, is the promise and the possibility; it is a man's capability for life for and *with* his fellow man, that is, it is the external basis of covenant . . ." ([25], p. 32). Love can make itself felt within this order of justice through the administration of *equity* in social arrangements, since equity considers particular neighbors' special needs for help and rescue. Equity considerations can also correct, improve, and humanize our property laws by reminding us of their very purpose. This is, then, in Ramsey's view, an example of "love-transformed-justice"[4]

The theme of love-transformed-justice throws a very positive light upon the created order of civil law and its functions in *Christian Ethics and the Sit-In*. But Ramsey also goes on to explicate the negative function of civil law and the State based upon God's *restraining* grace. For, "sin croucheth at the door" of all human communal life, and thus it is through coercive legal institutions that God intends to preserve "a tolerable fellow humanity against the ravagements of sin."[5] Because of this, "Christian realism" must temper its transformist zeal with a respect – a *very strong* respect – for the established order of law, "unless and until some better garment can be woven without letting worse befall" ([25], p. 48; see also [26], p. 124). The presumption here (and elsewhere) seems to be that "worse" generally *will* befall, except in unusual (and largely unspecified) cases. Indeed, Ramsey has been criticized over the years for seeming to elevate the 'preservative' concern for maintaining legal order too far above the 'creative' and 'redemptive' concerns of justice and love – especially in light of such statements as, ". . . in the Christian view, simple and not so simple injustice *alone* has never been sufficient justification for revolutionary change."[6] Charles Curran has claimed that, starting with *Christian Ethics and the Sit-In*, Ramsey treats order as a 'terminal value' along with justice (even love-transformed justice), and that his later treatises in just war theory and medical ethics give tremendous weight to the former value – just as those works tend to emphasize the restraint-of-sin function of civil law (at the expense of further, developed practical application of the love-transformed-justice motif in the political realm) ([9], esp. Chapter 1 and pp. 80–90, 105–109). At any rate, Ramsey himself has claimed explicitly only that order is not a higher value than justice and justice is not a higher value than order ([30], p. 11).

To move on, however, the motif of "love transforming justice" (or "Christ transforming the natural law") provides the central theme of another major work, *Nine Modern Moralists* (1962), in which Ramsey develops and explicates his "Protestant view of the natural law." Here is the culmination of a marked shift in emphasis from that of *Basic Christian Ethics*. The earlier volume, with its stress upon the neighbor-oriented freedom of *agape*, had "refused to locate natural law as belonging to the new that had come with Christ," although it had allowed that love might make use of ethical wisdom "from whatsoever source" in formulating social policy ([28], p. 6). *Nine Modern Moralists*, in contrast, focuses upon that "whatsoever source" of moral wisdom itself, whose norms of justice are permeable to elevation and transformation by love. Having established some ethical implications of God's 'ordering' work in creation in *Christian Ethics and the Sit-In* and *War and the Christian Conscience*, Ramsey now seeks to describe how such moral norms can be 'naturally' known. He continues to reject the 'traditional' Roman Catholic interpretation of natural law (as he understands it), involving rational deduction of moral norms from a static representation of humankind's universal and essential nature. Actually, the core of his complaint is that the rigidity and absolutism so often associated with natural law theory is the result of Catholics' claims that "revelation has 'republished' the entire natural law and thereby made our knowledge of it certain and exact" ([28], p. 212f.). Instead, Ramsey chooses to follow the lead of the revisionist Catholic theologian Jacques Maritain in claiming that natural justice is perceived not primarily through reason but rather through inclination. Its principles are discovered phenomenologically, through the evidence of experienced particulars, rather than through purely rational perception of ontological necessity. Thus, no human being natively possesses the content of the natural law itself; he acquires knowledge of it "in the course of active reflection upon man in the context of moral, social, and legal decisions" ([28], pp. 212, 216). Beginning with this insight, then, a Protestant doctrine of natural law would separate that notion from any ecclesiastical authority so that its inherent meaning can be fulfilled in ongoing discovery of new and relevant truth through the unlimited discussion of free persons ([28], pp. 229–30). And it is through this epistemological process that "a profound religious apprehension of human existence" may transform natural justice. Resorting again to Barthian language, Ramsey remarks that our knowledge of natural justice through fundamental inclination or disinclination provides the "external" basis and possibility for life in covenant; covenant-righteousness provides the "internal" basis or true meaning and purpose of our understanding of whatever we come to know of 'essential' human nature ([28], p. 244).

Ramsey's 'Yes' to this phenomenological interpretation of natural law is of tremendous significance for our understanding of his later, topical applications[7] of "covenant fidelity" as a *universal* ethical norm. For, his treatises on medical ethics are addressed not specifically to the Christian community but to the human community at large. He expects a "convergence" between religion and humanism at the level of particular moral judgements; and covenant-fidelity is presented as the meaning of both natural and revealed morality. In his Preface to *The Patient as Person*, for example, he begins with explicitly biblical language of "fidelity to covenant" and "righteousness," but then goes on to mix this language with non-religious synonyms:

I hold with Karl Barth that covenant-fidelity is the inner meaning and purpose of our creation as human beings, while the whole of creation is the external basis and condition of the possibility of covenant. This means that the conscious acceptance of covenant responsibilities is the inner meaning of even the 'natural' or systemic relations into which we are born and of the institutional relations or roles we enter by choice, while this fabric provides the external framework for human fulfillment in explicit covenants among men. The practice of medicine is one such covenant. *Justice, fairness, righteousness, canons of loyalty, the sanctity of life, hesed, agape* or *charity* are some of the names given to the moral quality of attitude and of action owed to all men by any man who steps into covenant with another man . . . ([32], pp. xii–xiii).

So, we cannot escape "*the* ethical question" of the meaning of *faithfulness*, because we all *do* exist in covenant relations, whether by nature, choice or need.[8]

For the most part, Ramsey's major works in medical ethics can, then, be described as reflections upon and analyses of the demands of covenant-faithfulness in the physician-patient or researcher-subject relationship. Interestingly, these demands turn out to be strikingly uni-directional. Although the term 'covenant' commonly implies *reciprocal* agreements, claims and responsibilities, Ramsey focuses almost entirely on what is owed *to* patients or research subjects *by* the professional, with little mention of anything owed (or available for offer) by the former groups. One obvious reason for this one-way emphasis is *agape*'s orientation toward the neighbor's *need*: the medical needs of patients are the foundational reason for most physician-patient relationships. But one might yet ask whether medical professionals do not have needs, claims or expectations which might also be addressed within a 'covenantal' understanding of medicine.[9]

It should be pointed out, too, that Ramsey's considerable contributions in the field of medical ethics have been largely polemical in nature. His continuing concern has been the moral *ethos* of our society and the level of our ongoing moral discourse. In *The Patient as Person*, for example, he seeks to protect the notion of man's "sacredness" in the biological order from the twin threats of medical vitalism and medical utilitarianism. In *Fabricated Man* [31] he seeks to preserve our understanding of the nature of human parenthood from the encroachment of end-oriented technological imperatives which might rend asunder the unitive and procreative aspects of sexual covenants. And his last major treatise on medical ethics, *Ethics at the Edges of Life* [41], is in large part an attempt, as James Childress puts it, to "clean up our moral and legal reasoning in order to sustain an ethos that provides the only real restraint against active, involuntary euthanasia" ([7], p. 182). Because his arguments are so often mounted against some other identifiable moral position, Ramsey's style of writing is frequently indignant and even bellicose. Moreover, his interpretations of covenant-fidelity's positive obligations are often expressed in negative or limiting terms, defining what we *ought not* to do to one another. He is fond of quoting Sir Derrick Dunlop, for instance: "The end does not always justify the means, and the good things that men do can be made complete only by the things they refuse to do" ([32], p. xiv; [31], p. 123). This assertion neatly summarizes Ramsey's rejection of any primarily teleological ethic; it also hints at his response to the question, "Are there some things we should *always* refuse to do?"

So, before proceeding to some of his substantive arguments in medical ethics, perhaps we should examine a bit further Ramsey's understanding of moral principles and rules, and the possibility of exceptionless moral rules.

2. PRINCIPLES, RULES, AND 'EXCEPTIONS' IN RAMSEY'S ETHICS

We have seen that the central, foundational norm in Ramsey's moral theory is *agape*, or covenant-love oriented toward meeting the neighbor's need. We have also seen that, as early as *Basic Christian Ethics*, with its emphasis on the freedom of *agape*, Ramsey was claiming that love might "use" binding moral rules from other epistemological sources to further its concrete social aims (provided that love remain the "controlling partner" in such alliances). His later terminological shifts to "in-principled love," "love-transformed-justice," and "covenant-fidelity" reflect the development of his notion of "Protestant natural law" as an independent source of moral norms alongside *agape*; these shifts also reflect his growing insistence upon the necessity of stability and continuity in moral life – the kind of consistency which requires recognition of stable moral norms. Indeed, Ramsey has always waged battle against theories of ethical relativism, particularly in Christian ethics, as they seem to him "always in peril of opening the floodgates of anarchy and license in the name of freedom from the law."[10]

Since this section is concerned with the sources and theoretical relatedness of moral action-guides in Ramsey's work, and with his views about exceptions to them, we would do well to focus here upon two of his writings which deal most clearly with these issues: *Deeds and Rules in Christian Ethics* (1967) and a 1968 article, "The Case of the Curious Exception" ([22], pp. 67–135).

In *Deeds and Rules* Ramsey describes his own position as a form of "mixed agapism" – a term used by William Frankena in typologizing love-based

CHAPTER THREE

theories of Christian ethics ([12], [13]) – because of the two different senses in which *agape* may be related to principles of moral conduct. First, there are norms governing acts or practices which are implicit in, or may be derived directly from, *agape* itself. This is the meaning of "in-principled love." For instance, certain "forms of steadfastness in responsibility and accountability one to another would seem to be the most likely inference from Christlike love . . ." ([29], p. 164). (One who argues that the intrinsic demands of *agape* are our *only* reliable source of moral guidance might be said to espouse "*pure* agapism.") But, second, there are also "structures of life into which we are called; and practices into which every man is born who ever was born," and the norms implicit in these "orders of creation" are also known to some extent through man's natural competence to make moral judgements. The 'mixture' of these two sources, *agape* and man's natural sense of justice/injustice, contains an "internal asymmetry" which is the meaning of "love transforming natural justice" ([29], pp. 120, 122, 164).

Frankena's typology of "agapism" had dealt not only with the epistemic sources of moral norms, however; it had also dealt with the weight or stringency of norms derived from these sources. His "pure act-agapism" would entail a 'situational' ethic of applying one's loving will to the 'facts' of the case in order to render only situation-specific judgements, with no overriding concern about traditionally-accepted moral norms which might be violated in the process. This type of agapism bears structural similarities to some other teleological theories of morality in that it focuses upon producing good ends or consequences (as required, in this case, by love for the neighbor). "Summary rule-agapism" would identify "working rules" of practice as generally love-embodying and to be followed unless doing so seems to contradict what love requires in a particular context. "Pure rule-agapism," on the other hand, would entail *consistently* following rules of practice *because* they are understood to be love-embodying. (A fourth 'type' would be a mixed theory, combining the former two or latter two approaches [12].)

Taking into account both bases of Frankena's typology of "agapism," Ramsey goes on to specify his own approach as "mixed rule-agapism." For, while he says that our experience of the claims of God's righteous love may allow some room for act-agapism, nevertheless it contains "an inward pressure toward rule-agapism" ([29], p. 48). *Agape* defines what is "right, righteous, [and] obligatory to be done among men" (as we noted earlier), and it is thus not simply a matter of choosing and doing the good as one perceives it in each unique situation of choice. A Christian "will be careful lest for 'what love directly requires' he has put 'what love (or sentiment) *immediately* requires'; and he knows that such unruly behavior may not be what love requires" ([29], p. 112).

Ramsey concludes, then, that if "agapism" is not a distinctive third type of moral theory alongside "teleology" and "deontology" (as Frankena had suggested it might be), then "it seems to me more true to say it is a type of deontology than to say that it is a type of teleology" ([29], p. 108). It must be noted, though, that a genuine dialectical tension does remain in his argument, as he claims to have shown

... that a proper understanding of the moral life will be one in which Christians determine what we ought to do in very great measure by determining which rules of action are most love-embodying, *but* that there are *also* always situations in which we are to tell what we should do by getting clear about the facts of that situation and then asking what is the loving or the most loving thing to do in it ([29], p. 5, emphasis added).

It is also true, however, that Ramsey's analyses of concrete ethical issues consistently emphasize a rule-dominant moral approach. And the next critical question he goes on to consider is whether we should view our moral action-guides as mere "summaries" of past wisdom (about actions which are love-embodying) and open to possible future exceptions, or whether there are "general rules of practices"[11] which *define* what is always love-fulfilling in particular circumstances and which are thus constantly applicable and not exceptable on direct appeal to *agape*. In Ramsey's view of the matter, reflection upon "summary rules" offers at least two good reasons for moving toward acceptance of binding "general" rules. First, an agent's direct application of *agape* to his own particular case affords a greater likelihood of "making a mistake" than if he follows a rule applicable to his case. And, second, exceptional actions (which may seem most loving in light of their *direct* consequences) may *indirectly* tend to break down the social practice of behavioral rules which are generally love-embodying ([29, p. 126).

Moreover, Ramsey is convinced that Christian faith and love offers us more than just "probable knowledge" about the significance of binding moral rules:

A position we might call 'pure or general rule-agapism' would seem to be entailed in any conviction that in Jesus Christ the righteousness of God and the mystery of the ages, the meaning of the creation, of mature manhood, and the destination of man toward unfailing covenant with God and with fellowman, have been made manifest. An unbinding love would seem the least likely conclusion one would reach if he seriously regarded the freedom of God's love in binding Himself to the world as the model for all covenants between men. Could anyone who perceives that God in total love and total freedom bound Himself to the world possibly view the implications of this love as unbinding on men? ([29], p. 127f.)

Thus, reflection on the realities of moral community and a full appreciation of God's covenant-making love both support the conclusion that general rules are consistent with the "freedom of *agape*" – that we can and should recognize some things that are "as unconditionally wrong as love is unconditionally right" ([29], p. 129).

Such a claim presages Ramsey's answer to the query, "Are there some moral rules which should be closed to possible exceptions?" And he devotes considerable attention to that question in "The Case of the Curious Exception."

He begins that article by distinguishing, for the first time in his work, between moral "principles" and moral "rules." (Previously, he tells us, he had used the word "rule" to mean also "principle," "orders," "ordinances," "direction," and so on.) Here, "principles" are defined as general "*directions* of action"; "rules" are relatively more specific "*directives* of an action, prescribing or proscribing a *definite* action" and devolving from a broader principle ([22], p. 72f.).

He allows that his previous arguments for unexceptionable "rules" had really been concerned with generic "principles" (in the new terminology). And he goes on to offer yet another, formal reason for saying that some principles may be without exceptions. Specifically, when we offer moral justification for "exceptional" acts – that is, exemptions from the claims of a moral action-guide – we are also claiming justification for all other acts with the same kind of repeatable moral features (because of the requirement that moral judgements be universalizable). What we are really doing in such cases, then, is simply recognizing a new and nuanced *application* of (or *rule* deduced from) our original principle. Such a so-called "exception" is actually

... a deed falling within our deepened or broadened or more specific principles. It is a *sort* of thing, if justifiable. It is no unique or singular exception ([22], p. 82).

By way of illustration, Ramsey reflects upon Joseph Fletcher's case of Mrs. Bergmeier,[12] who managed to become impregnated by a guard in order to gain release from a Russian work camp and return to her bereft family. While her action might be described initially as a violation of the rule against extramarital sex (as an application of marital fidelity), Ramsey suggests that her situation enabled her "to make explicit certain meanings and stipulations that were all along *implicit* in the meaning of *marital fidelity*" ([22], p. 87). After all, her ostensible justification for her deed was the restoration of "the bond between love-giving and the transmission of fully human lives in the unity of [her] family."[13] So, we might define it more accurately as an appropriate response to the faithfulness-claims of her marriage rather than as the meaning of the forbidden "adultery."

However, even if justifiable "exceptions" to some general *principles* are really only clarified and deepened applications of them, we may yet ask whether there are also any specific "definite-action *rules*" which should be understood as exceptionless. Here again, Ramsey believes that there certainly are such rules, and that the case is strongest for some social "rules of practice" and for "person-centered" rules of faithfulness to one's fellowmen. His reasons for strengthening rules of practice are essentially the same as he gave in *Deeds and Rules*: Such rules should be closed to further qualification if doing so decreases the likelihood of one's making a moral mistake, or if holding them open to future possible exceptions might indirectly promote general wrongdoing.[14]

Further, with respect to person-centered rules of faithfulness (or "canons of loyalty") he insists that, since human covenants are patterned after God's steadfast and faithful covenant-keeping, it follows that Christians should be "enormously disinterested" in locating rule-exceptions justified by possible future consequence-features or by consequence-oriented imaginary cases. Instead, we are driven to examine more deeply the meanings of covenant-obligation in order to recognize the *faithfulness*-exhibiting features of acts, relations, or situations. And, to leave our canons of loyalty open to consequence-based future qualification "would be to place fidelity in peril" ([22], pp. 125–27).

In closing his lengthy argument, Ramsey offers several examples of fidelity-based rules which, in his view, should most certainly be held closed to possible future exceptions. These include: do not rape (i.e., force sexual intercourse on an unwilling person); never involve a human subject in medical experimentation without his voluntary, informed consent; do not sterilize poor women as a condition for their receiving public assistance or child-support; and never directly attack non-combatant persons in warfare (i.e., the rule of discrimination or non-combatant immunity).[15] In all of these examples, the most apparent possible grounds for exception-making in particular (or hypothetical) cases would be appeals to the positive consequences of allowing some exceptions. But Ramsey's point here, as always, is that consequence-considerations, while admittedly important, must be secondary to our steadfast and consistent obligations of covenant-loyalty.[16]

We have seen, then, that Ramsey's ethic of covenant-fidelity (which he equates with an ethic of *agape*) involves an approach to moral decision-making contrasting sharply with McCormick's teleology of value-realization. The two moralists differ, for instance, on the central and controlling focus of Christian morality (covenant-obedience vs. realization of ordered values), on the epistemological grounding of natural law precepts (experiential-phenomenological vs. "prediscursively" perceived), and, practically, on the relative weight of consequence-considerations in moral judgement. These differences and others will be illustrated more clearly in the remaining three sections of this chapter, as we examine Ramsey's views on concrete medico-moral dilemmas.

3. DEFECTIVE NEWBORNS AND "MEDICAL INDICATIONS"

In Ramsey's view, morally proper treatment decisions in neonatology must systematically exclude even the minimal sort of quality-of-life criteria advocated by McCormick. For, the very notion of 'quality of life' assessments is, as he sees it, denied by the "equality of life" implicit in *agape*. Moral reflection upon treatment must instead focus on two foundational notions: the equal and independent value (sanctity) of each human life; and the "care" demanded by covenant-fidelity in a medical context.

To begin, as we did in the previous chapter, with theological assessments of the meaning of death, it is clear that Ramsey's attitude or perspective in dealing with it is somewhat more negative than McCormick's. Both thinkers affirm the existential fearsomeness of death; on the other hand, both also affirm in some sense the Christian confidence that death does not spell our ultimate separation from God. The difference between them, then, is largely one of emphasis or degree; but the attitudinal contrast is profound, nonetheless. We have seen, for instance, that McCormick views human physical life as *a* good foundational for the attainment of other values, which are themselves oriented toward our *summum bonum* (which transcends physical life and death). Ramsey, on the other hand, flatly rejects any description of life as "*a* good." Rather, he says, whenever we speak of *good* in any sense "we speak of *life's* well-being" ([41], p. 207). For this reason, Ramsey believes McCormick's theory of "proportionate reason" to be flawed at its very foundations, since the value of life is "incommensurable" with other goods against which it might be 'weighed' (see [42]).

Undergirding this incommensurability thesis is Ramsey's firm rejection of what he calls the theological-anthropological "mistake" of Platonic/Cartesian dualism of body and soul. The human person must be considered "a sacredness in bodily life . . . He is an embodied soul or an ensouled body"; he is certainly *not* a soul endowed with the capacity to "wear out and outlast his body" ([32], p. xiii; [35], p. 60 – emphasis added). Indeed, Ramsey's understanding of both Scripture and tradition leads him to assert emphatically that, "for Biblical or later Christian anthropology, the only possible form which human life in any true and proper sense can take *here or hereafter* is 'somatic'" ([27], p. 3). Within this anthropology, death was and is and will remain an "enemy" or "alien power." Ramsey accepts the Pauline symbolism of death as "a conquered enemy, to be accepted in the name of the Conqueror," but insists nevertheless that it is "an enemy, surely, and not simply an acceptable part of the natural order of things" ([35], pp. 51, 57).

There is, of course, no little ambiguity in conceiving of death as at once an enemy to be dreaded and a "conquered" enemy. This ambiguity – or paradox – is maintained (and even sharpened) rather than being resolved in Ramsey's writings. One reason for this is that most of his more recent reflections upon the concept of death have appeared in writings which are issue-specific and polemical. In his chapter in *The Patient as Person* entitled "On (Only) Caring for the Dying," Ramsey inveighs against excessive medical vitalism toward the dying by reminding us that "Christians believe that death and dying are a *part of life* and like birth *no less a gift of God* . . ." and that "the dying cannot pass beyond God's love and care" ([32], pp. 153, 156–57 – emphasis added). On the other hand, his most extensive conceptual treatment of death appears in two 1974 articles ([35], [36]) concerned with rebutting the presumptions of the 'death with dignity' movement and the pro-euthanasia ethos he sees as its logical outcome. And here he points approvingly to the "ancient recipe" that "death is *not a part of life*"; there can be dignity and nobility in caring for the dying, "but not in dying itself" ([35], p. 50). He amends his earlier death-as-gift metaphor somewhat by insisting that, "I know of no Christian teaching that assures us that our 'final end' is 'equally' beautiful as birth, growth and fulness of life. Moreover, if revelation disclosed any such thing it would be contrary to reason and to the human reality and experience of death."[17]

As Ramsey sees it, the Christian understanding of the event of death correlates closely with its understanding in a "true humanism," so his emphasis in both 1974 articles is upon the existential "awfulness and awefullness of death itself" ([36], p. 502). Reflecting on Stewart Alsop's memoir of terminal illness, *Stay of Execution*, Ramsey observes that one's death ". . . cannot fail to be for him an irreparable loss, an unquenchable grief, the threat of all threats, a dread that is more than all fears aggregated together, an approaching 'evil' which annuls every ordinary distinction between good and evil . . ." ([36], p. 501).

The final thrust of both articles, however, is not simply the horror of death but rather what that horror teaches us about the sanctity (or dignity) of *life*. In short, "The more 'life' (unique, individual life) becomes a pro-word, the more death is an enemy; the more death is an anti-word, the more pro we should be and will be in respect for any of our companions in this dying life of ours." Human persons are of non-interchangeable, unrepeatable significance. A denial of death's indignity would require also a refusal of personal worth and uniqueness. And *that*, in Ramsey's view, would spell the end of "intensive *care*" for dying persons ([36], p. 502). These later theological-anthropological (and 'humanistic') assertions about the meaning of death serve, then, to buttress Ramsey's earlier arguments (e.g., in *The Patient as Person*) about our obligations to respect others as "a sacredness in their bodily lives" and to provide medical 'care' as a fulfillment of covenant-fidelity. Both obligations are, for Ramsey, immediately derivative of *agape*, but should also be clear to "any man who steps into a covenant [such as that between health professional and patient] with another man."[18]

Respect for life's sanctity debars any evaluative consideration of its *quality*, on Ramsey's terms. All human lives are of "equal and independent value," and comparative quality-of-life judgements deny that essential equality. Our standard should be God's attitude toward us: "Our God is no respector of persons of good quality. Nor does he curtail his care for us because our parents are poor or have unhappy marriages, or because we are most in need of help." Indeed, God has "special care for the weak and the vulnerable . . . He cares according to *need*, not capacity or merit" ([41], pp. 203, 205 – emphasis added). In our medical treatment decisions, then, we should "play God as God plays God" – i.e., we should care for the sick and dying by meeting their individual medical (i.e., physiological) needs.

This normative definition of medical "agent care" does not always entail aggressive treatment, however. Where care in the form of *cure* is not possible, it cannot be morally required, and it gives place to care in the form of comfort for the dying: "[C]are means always hoping to cure and to save life until that becomes, in the case of the dying, useless; and care means always abiding with the dying patient until that becomes useless" ([41], p. 219, n. 43). The key descriptive term here is "dying": concrete moral obligations of care are altered when the patient enters irreversibly into "the dying process."

Here we have the fundamentals of Ramsey's treatment policy for defective newborns (and all other incompetent patients, including the terminally ill): those treatments are morally required which are "medically indicated." Applied to the 'Baby Doe' cases mentioned in Chapter 1, for example, surgical treatment of a Down's baby is morally required because it is not "useless" and is medically indicated. Retardation and other handicaps are morally irrelevant because they do not prevent the babies' survival (if they are surgically treated). To treat these babies as if they were 'dying', or to withhold treatment because of the diminished 'quality' of their prospective lives, would be an "abandonment" of agent-care. Ramsey praises McCormick's unwillingness to base treatment decisions on the quality of the patient's "external" conditions (such as poverty, family status, etc.), but he argues that McCormick has not gone far enough. For, "[i]t is hard to see how conditions external to the individual and 'the very condition of the individual' can be kept as distinct as McCormick, admirably, tries to keep them" ([41], p. 175). Indeed, Ramsey is very much concerned about the current social ethos regarding 'quality of life' and the logical entailments he fears will flow from it:

If intensive care of defective newborns should, at a point, cease because of expected quality of life, how can we avoid also concluding that a pediatrician's 'intensive care for the 1200 gm offspring of the 13-year-old unmarried girl from the ghetto' ought also to cease? ([41], p. 176).

The moral solution to all possible inequalities or misapplications of a 'quality of life' standard is, then, a "medical indications policy." And such a policy establishes a moral rule of "giving equally vigorous treatment to defective newborns as to normals."

Clearly, Ramsey's emphasis is not on the procedural issue of *who* makes treatment decisions for defective infants; he is instead concerned with the *content* of such decisions. A medical indications policy considers only the 'objective' details of the patient's medical condition, not the possibly 'subjective' personal values of family or physician which might color assessments of the infant's 'best interests':

> The tests for telling whether to discontinue treatments should be clinical or physiological ones . . . , not anyone's 'values.' They should not *in themselves*, with or without intention, build into the conditions for allowing the dying to die a discriminatory definition of a life worth living. A fortiori, *whoever decides* these questions should not be able to give effect to his own 'values' in this regard as if they were certainly the patient's own ([43], p. 133).

In terms of public policy, this view does not inherently prescribe any particular decision-making priority among families, physicians, or courts – so long as the 'right' decision is made for the right reasons.[19] For all practical purposes, however, primary responsibility for decision-making apparently would rest with the person most capable of assessing 'medical indications' – namely, the attending physician. It is hardly surprising, then, that Ramsey devotes so much of his attention to the physician's particular covenant-obligations of agent-care.

He admits, though, that there are cases of dying patients who are *beyond* care – that is, beyond both cure and comfort. In *The Patient as Person* he describes two possible patient-groups who may suggest "qualifications" of our duty always to care: those "irretrievably inaccessible to human care" because they are deeply and permanently comatose; and those in "indefeatable agony" whose pain cannot be kept at bay ([32], pp. 161–64). In these rare cases (and *only* in these cases) Ramsey allows that even "assisted dying" may be justifiable, that "the crucial moral difference between omission and commission . . . has utterly vanished."[20] Later, in *Ethics at the Edges of Life*, he suggests caveats to this earlier "venture into exception-making." He does not recant his moral justification of some individual *acts* of dispatch, but questions whether any such *rule of practice* should ever be recognized, because

> . . . for whole teams of the caring profession (physicians, nurses, interns, medical students) to begin to induce death as a practice would be one more step in the erosion of the moral distinction between voluntary and involuntary euthanasia and between allowing to die and direct killing ([41], p. 216).

Furthermore, allowing exceptions for patients in insurmountable pain "might too readily become an excuse for bad medical management of pain." Given these considerations, then, Ramsey opts for an unexceptionable rule of practice proscribing euthanasia, while yet holding that courageous conscientious objection to it may be warranted for some physicians in particular cases ([41], p. 217).

In practical terms, Ramsey's "medical indications policy" depends almost entirely upon which prognostic category a particular patient might fit into – e.g., "incurable non-dying" vs. "dying". Only for the [incompetent or comatose] patient who is already "in the dying process" (that is, one for whom death is "impending and imminent" and for whom any attempt at cure would be "useless") does Ramsey find it morally appropriate, as an expression of agent-care, to cease curative efforts.

However, the determination that a given patient has in fact reached the "onset of the process of dying" – a judgement Ramsey repeatedly tells us can be made only by the physician – is surely not so neat and simple as he assumes. Take, for example, the well-known case of Karen Ann Quinlan, who died (of untreated pneumonia) on June 11, 1985, ten years after she had lapsed into a persistent vegetative state and nine years after the New Jersey Supreme Court granted her parents permission to remove her respirator. Ramsey criticized that court's decision (and the lower court decision which it reversed) for relying on some standard other than a medical indications policy ([41], pp. 268–99). He implied that the matter of removing the respirator should have been morally obvious, since Karen was "clearly dying."[21] And he even went so far as to point out the moral difference between "returning [Karen] to her natural state of impending death" (justifiable) and withholding life-sustaining, indicated medical treatment from a "nondying" patient simply because her "natural state . . . means *noncognitivity* or incurability" (unjustifiable) ([41], p. 285). But what are we to say about this sort of distinction in Karen's case? By the time Ramsey's reflections were published in *Ethics at the Edges of Life* (1978), she had been ventilator-independent for nearly two years and gave no indication of imminent demise. She was in many respects physically healthy, albeit non-conscious. It would seem, then, given Ramsey's own descriptive distinctions, that Karen's prognostic status could be described more accurately as "noncognitive, incurable, nondying." She had, of course, reached the point where no treatment would be "useful" in treating her *noncognitivity*, but that condition was not causing (and did not cause) her death. Yet Ramsey, while insisting that "value-judgements" about noncognitivity or any other "measure of the 'less than human'" should never be the basis for treatment choices, was still willing to describe her as "dying" and to view removal of her respirator as "medically indicated."

Further complicating this all-important descriptive muddle is Ramsey's earlier proposal (in *The Patient as Person*) of those two possible classes of "dying" patients, "irretrievably inaccessible to human care," for whom "assisted dying" might be justifiable. One of those classes includes those "in deep and irreversible coma who can be and are maintained alive for many, many years." Such patients feel no suffering and would not feel hunger if nourishment were withheld. It is then "a matter of complete indifference whether death gains the victory over the patient in such impenetrable solitude by direct or indirect action" ([32], p. 162). Now, for all intents and purposes Karen Quinlan fit *this* description, too. From the various news accounts of her case, it would not seem inconsistent for her physicians to have described her condition as at once "terminally comatose but not immediately dying" *and* "irretrievably inaccessible to human care" – even as Professor Ramsey's reflections on her case were being published. And this possible (indeed, probable) ambiguity in categorizing her *condition* would, on Ramsey's analysis of covenant-obligations, lead to a correlative ambiguity in determining morally required treatment (or morally justifiable nontreatment, or even "assisted death") in her case. Granted, Ramsey has *stipulated* that irreversible coma (or persistent vegetative state) is equivalent to "dying" for purposes of morally assessing treatment decisions, on the grounds that persons in that condition are "inaccessible to human care." But is not such a stipulation also tacit acceptance of at least a minimal "quality of life" criterion – i.e., consciousness? (I will return to this question in Chapter 6.) Surely Karen Quinlan's case illustrates the tenuousness of equating permanent unconsciousness with "dying" in terms of actual *medical* prognoses.

There are, too, cases involving defective newborns that both expand and challenge the precision of "incurable nondying" vs. "dying" distinctions. Ramsey himself points to the case of the anencephalic newborn as one who is not even born "alive" in terms of his/her physiological integrity, who is thus utterly inaccessible to our care, and who should therefore be given only respect "like the respect to be given to the corpse of a deceased" ([41], pp. 212–14). But there is another sort of case of a "nondying" infant who, in Ramsey's view, might nevertheless belong to that class of patients totally inaccessible to our care because of "insurmountable pain." These infants are afflicted with Lesch-Nyhan Syndrome, a genetic condition transmitted only to males and which causes physical and mental retardation, spastic cerebral palsy, and compulsive self-mutilation. As soon as the infant cuts teeth, he compulsively gnaws through lip, fingers, toes, and other body parts. Once this process begins, Ramsey tells us, the infant is probably in insurmountable agony and "beyond human caring action." And since *palliative* care is then (by definition) impossible, it may be that even the moral significance of distinguishing between constant care and direct dispatch is lost.[22]

What we might ask of Ramsey at this point, however, is, What about the extent of our obligation to care *before* the onset of self-mutilation? Most cases of Lesch-Nyhan are not actually diagnosed until the onset of symptoms; and Ramsey confines his discussion to the symptomatic period. But diagnosis is possible even before birth (by amniocentesis).[23] So let us consider the hypothetical case of a Lesch-Nyhan child diagnosed at some point *before* the self-mutilating stage. Ramsey's discussion would seem to imply two different treatment prescriptions during that pre-symptomatic period. On the one hand, he has introduced both anencephaly and Lesch-Nyhan cases as possible "*exceptions* to the principle of giving equally vigorous treatment to defective newborns as to normals." And one might reasonably infer from this that he would prescribe only palliative forms of care before symptom-manifestation (in anticipation of that awful onset). On the other hand, though, the child *is* "accessible to our care" in this pre-symptomatic period, and is not "in the dying process" until long after the onset of symptoms. Further, Ramsey is consistently averse to basing treatment decisions on measurements of *how much* 'quality-time' a patient might have left. And this would seem to imply an obligation to treat maximally and vigorously any medical problems occurring in the pre-symptomatic period.

So, to sharpen the question raised by our hypothetical case, let us assume further that our pre-symptomatic Lesch-Nyhan baby also has a congenital heart defect inconsistent with survival for more than a few months unless repaired immediately. Should he be subjected to the surgery (or surgeries)? Unless Ramsey is prepared to 'draw a line' by claiming that there is some definable point at which the baby suddenly becomes "inaccessible to our care," it would appear that his message – at least as it concerns care in the pre-symptomatic period – remains a mixed one at best.

We might raise the same sort of situational question about Tay-Sachs babies. These children are born with an incurable inborn error in lipid metabolism resulting in gradual accumulation of a chemical (ganglioside GM_2) in their brains. Symptoms become manifest at about 6 months of age and include progressive dementia, blindness, paralysis, and finally death, usually by age 3 to 4 years. (Like Lesch-Nyhan Syndrome, Tay-Sachs Disease can be diagnosed even before birth, but often is not diagnosed until its symptoms appear.) Ramsey points out, though, that unlike Lesch-Nyhan babies, Tay-Sachs children are "accessible to our care" even in their dying (– the "onset" of which he places at approximately the onset of their symptoms). Treatment during that period need not include means which only *prolong* the dying process; palliative care is all that is required morally. However, he claims, with respect to the pre-symptomatic period, that "there is no reason for saying those six months are a life span of lesser worth to God than living seventy years before the onset of irreversible degeneration" ([41], p. 191). The implication of this is that treatment decisions for a Tay-Sachs child (during those six months) should reflect whatever would be chosen for a child without that genetic problem.

So let us consider a hypothetical Tay-Sachs case paralleling the above Lesch-Nyhan case (i.e., a diagnosed but pre-symptomatic baby with a life-threatening heart defect). Should we subject such a child to surgical interventions? If the child were otherwise healthy and 'normal' we would (and should) readily agree to the infant's surgery (or series of surgeries) – even if we could anticipate those invasive procedures requiring a 6- or 8-month recovery period. The same decision would apparently be required for our Tay-Sachs baby, in Ramsey's view of the matter.

Now, there are those who would recoil at this conclusion and would argue that we would best 'benefit' the child by simply keeping him pain-free while he dies of cardiac failure (thus intending to spare him the discomfort of invasive surgery followed immediately by the horrible onset of his disease process). Ramsey replies, though, that positive commandments to 'benefit' do not apply as stringently as negative ones like 'do no harm' – and he sees non-treatment as a 'harm' in a case like this ([41], p. 239). Of course, some would object that the surgery itself, coupled with the predictable degeneration to follow, might be seen as a 'harm' to be avoided on the child's behalf. To this objection Ramsey retorts (characteristically) that, compared to such an interpretation,

> ... all previous medical violations of the principle of 'do no harm,' all fallings short of a physician's covenant with his patient, all other departures from the *equality* of particular lives regardless of their state or condition, every past weakening of humanistic ethics, and all past atheisms that lost hold of the awesome claims of a human life and tried to rise above good and evil – all look puny by comparison ([41], p. 241).

In other words, Ramsey disagrees. 'Do no harm' can never be fulfilled, in his view, by allowing a 'nondying' infant to die.

There is, however, another consideration mentioned by Ramsey which might be relevant to the heart-defective Tay-Sachs (or Lesch-Nyhan) cases under scrutiny here. For, while Ramsey insists that we not compare patient-persons themselves (in terms of quality of life), he is somewhat open to comparison of *treatments*. He gives qualified approval to Warren Reich's claim that certain *circumstances* may make particular treatments themselves unacceptably burdensome. As Reich puts it, ". . . when the very means of effort to sustain life inseparably involves a truly grave excessive hardship, the obligation to continue may diminish to the point where one is no longer obliged to continue the efforts."[24] Ramsey's interpretation of this (applied to 'nondying' babies, as in the case at hand) is that "care and comfort should be chosen . . . for the nondying instead of burdensome treatments that themselves *diminish* the patient's reception of care and comfort and a human presence" ([41], p. 181 – emphasis added). Whether or not a series of invasive medical procedures would "diminish the reception of care and comfort" by a pre-symptomatic Tay-Sachs or Lesch-Nyhan child is, frankly, a rather conjectural (and, to some, inherently *qualitative*) medical judgement. But it is perhaps no more conjectural than the judgement that a particular patient has or has not crossed the line from the "incurable nondying" stage to the "onset of the dying process."

In defense of Ramsey's position, it must be said that it is generally clear (theoretically) and tightly argued. Some have questioned the consistency of its various logical entailments (e.g., Ramsey's suggestion that his "agent-morality" of covenant-care "ceases" when the care cannot be "received" by the patient-subject).[25] But certainly Ramsey cannot be accused of carelessness in his reasoning about covenant-obligations in medicine. The questions raised in the last few pages have instead centered upon the 'factual' element in his moral reasoning. Are his neat conceptual distinctions between "incurable nondying" and "dying," or between "accessible to care" and "inaccessible to care," really that clear and/or useful on the wards? Furthermore, many of us who have worked in patient-care settings (and especially in care for the terminally ill) are aware that the phrase "medically indicated" is actually *employed* quite often in ways which seem to suggest a broader range of considerations than simply physiological status and/or prospects.[26] And it is this very awareness which has led some commentators – McCormick, for instance – to argue that such language masks or presupposes value-judgements about the patient's condition, judgements whose *moral* validity should be discursively analyzed and evaluated toward the end of determining at least minimal standards for what patient-conditions are "reasonably" sustained. Actual "common usage" is surely an important factor to consider when employing any term or phrase *normatively*, and perhaps Ramsey could have avoided some (unintentional) unclarities if he had chosen some other terminology to express unequivocally what *he* means.

4. MEDICAL INDICATIONS AND PATIENT AUTONOMY

As we have seen, a patient's prognostic status makes all the difference for Ramsey when it comes to treatment choices for the voiceless. And one of his other supporting reasons for so limiting the range of proxy decisions, in addition to those noted thus far, is that we cannot *know*, in the case of a never-competent patient, what that patient *would* choose if (s)he were capable of choosing. So let us turn now to Ramsey's views about treatment decisions made *by* fully competent patients for themselves – particularly in terms of the patient's 'right to refuse treatment.' Since those views have undergone a significant shift in emphasis over time, it will be necessary at the outset to deal with them chronologically.

In Chapter 3 of *The Patient as Person* Ramsey explores and 'updates' the moral import of the traditional 'ordinary' vs. 'extraordinary' treatments distinction. In his view, the first leg of that distinction – the 'prospect of benefit' factor – has direct moral application to the irreversibly dying: "There is no obligation to do anything that is useless" ([32], p. 127). Where cure is impossible, covenant-fidelity requires "(only) caring for the dying." He goes on to suggest, further, that the traditional distinction's second leg – the calculus of benefit/hardship for the patient – may offer other good moral grounds for withholding or discontinuing treatment:

The 'process of dying' is not the only condition for stopping the use of medical means, although when present it is a sufficient and morally obliging condition. Other conditions can make it morally right to stop the use of medical means, although the decision to do so may not be a strictly medical judgement . . .

. . . Even when he could succeed [medically], a doctor may and sometimes should allow his medical judgement to defer to a patient's estimate of the higher importance of the worth and the relations for which his life was lived ([32], p. 136f.).

Significantly, Ramsey confines his attention to the *physician's* role or perspective, even while describing the patient's own "good moral reasons" for rejecting life-prolonging treatment. But he does not shrink from suggesting examples of patient-reasons that a "humane wisdom" would accept. He agrees with some of the Catholic manualists of earlier centuries, for instance, that one might reasonably choose to die (sooner) among family and friends than to travel great distances for treatment; or one might reject life-preserving surgery because of the "human difficulty" of living with its deforming and painful consequences. In sum,

> Not every means for prolonging life, once it is successful and made available – even 'customary' medical practice – becomes thereby ordinary and mandatory upon both patient and doctor. There are always broader human factors to be taken into account, and these always in Christian medical ethics kept the saving of life from being made an absolute and inflexible norm, a hardship inhumanly applied ([32], p. 141).

Five years after the publication of *The Patient as Person*, Ramsey delivered the Bampton Lectures in America, entitled "Christian Ethics and Modern Medicine." One of those lectures, published in 1977 as " 'Euthanasia' and Dying Well Enough," [40] takes up once again the notions of 'ordinary' and 'extraordinary' means of treatment. This time, however, Ramsey urges that we abandon the traditional terminology (because of what those terms are often mistakenly assumed to mean) and goes on to suggest that the distinction's morally significant meaning can be reduced "almost without remainder" to two components: 1) a comparison of medically indicated or not indicated treatments; and 2) "a patient's right to refuse treatment" ([40], p. 44). Having stated the matter in this way, though, he adds a caveat to his own second component: the patient's freedom and dignity "do not encompass the right . . . to assault the value of his own life *with medical assistance*" ([40], p. 45 – emphasis added). Ramsey's overarching concern here is to avoid any definitional leap from a 'right to refuse treatment' to a 'right to die,' since the latter right would logically entail (in his view) a correlative duty upon others to actively *assist* in the patient's dying, if requested. And the practice of such assistance would be violative of the covenant-based requirements of medical care.

This same article was much revised and included in *Ethics at the Edges of Life* (1978). In its revised form, Ramsey begins by reviewing five possible (but not mutually exclusive) standards for determining morally when to withhold or withdraw medical treatment: 1) the traditional ordinary/extraordinary means distinction; 2) a standard-medical-care policy; 3) a patient's right to refuse treatment; 4) a medical indications policy; and 5) a quality-of-expected-life policy. But now he argues that "the morally significant meaning of these similar and related standards can be reduced *almost without remainder to a medical indications policy*" ([41], p. 155). As if his shift in emphasis were not clear enough in that statement, he then proceeds to attack rhetorically his own earlier formulation of the matter:

> Why not say that the classification 'ordinary/extraordinary' can simply be reduced to (1) a determination either of the treatment indicated or that there is not treatment indicated in the

case of the dying, and (2) a patient's right to refuse treatment? The answer to that question is that there are medically indicated treatments (these used to be called 'ordinary') that a competent conscious patient has *no right to refuse*, just as no one has a moral right deliberately to ruin his health. Treatment refusal is a *relative right*, contrary to what is believed today by those who would reduce medical ethics to patient autonomy and a 'right to die.'

... A medical indications policy is applicable both to the non-dying and to the dying, to the conscious and the unconscious. Instead of a conscious nondying patient's right to refuse treatment we need to emphasize his free and informed *participation* in medical decisions affecting him when there are alternative treatments ([41], p. 156 – emphasis added).

This comprises Ramsey's latest and most emphatic statement concerning autonomous treatment refusals. He is still concerned to avoid the logical entailment of death-assistance which he associates with a 'right to die,' but he also seems to be asserting at least a presumptive *duty* of 'nondying' (though incurable) patients to remain that way as long as possible. His earlier caveat to a 'right to refuse treatment' is now amended to say that the patient's freedom and dignity "do not encompass the right ... to assault the value of his own life *with or without medical assistance*" ([41], p. 158 – emphasis added).

The most readily apparent reason for this shift in emphasis is that Ramsey's purpose in *Ethics at the Edges* is to correct what he considers a dangerous drift in our social ethos toward acceptance of both voluntary euthanasia and the nonvoluntary euthanasia of 'defective' patients. Specifically, he fears that acceptance of any standard other than a medical indications policy as 'reasonable' grounds for autonomous treatment-refusal by the non-dying might also be projected onto the incompetent or unconscious nondying as a reasonable presumption of *their* wishes or 'best interests.'

Beyond this fear, however, are more fundamental reasons for rejecting a full-fledged right of autonomous treatment-refusal. Ramsey believes we have but two alternatives with respect to death: "dying well enough," or choosing death as an end or means ([41], p. 149). The latter alternative is simply wrong, in his view, because of "our religious faith that life is a *gift*." To choose death as an end is to "throw the gift back in the face of the giver" ([41], p. 146).[27] Further, life is also a *trust*; we are not owners but stewards of our lives. "What, then, does one choose in a medical-moral policy of allowing to die or refusing further treatment – if that is not dominion (or co-dominion) over human life instead of trusteeship or stewardship, if that is not based on a fundamental denial that life is a gift and a trust?" ([41], p. 147).

Now, the language of 'gift' and 'trust' is simply a variation on Ramsey's usual references to 'covenant' and its obligations. But the issue here is not one of covenant-fidelity in the provision of medical care. Rather, Ramsey is describing a different sort of covenant-obligation: a duty of faithfulness owed *by* the patient *to* the Giver of Life. And he is not arguing that every nondying patient's refusal of further treatment is morally wrong, but only those refusals which constitute a choice *for death* as end or means. This was, he insists, the real wisdom of the traditional (ordinary/extraordinary means) distinction: it offered a way of referring to treatment refusals which are "simply suicidal" (and thus morally wrong) and those which are not. Recalling his *Patient as Person* examples of incurable patients who chose against disfiguring surgery or leaving home for treatment in a faraway place, he notes that these "were all *life* choices; none a choice of death as end or means" ([41], p. 157). Curiously, though, he now mitigates his earlier approval of even these choices by reminding us that medical progress has made many previously-extraordinary treatments not only 'ordinary' but "surely medically indicated and desirable." Moreover, he says, even choices for "dying well enough" may entail some sort of obligation of *assistance* from family or friends – and that is a negative moral factor not to be taken lightly in any treatment-refusal decision ([41], p. 156). In sum, Ramsey's emphasis upon the primacy of medical indications makes it most difficult to discern just *which* treatment refusals by the nondying (if any) he might now consider morally appropriate – even though he still allows that "a conscious, competent, 'incurable' patient would have a relative right to refuse treatment in the course of shared decision-making concerning his or her case" ([41], p. 165).

Despite its ambiguities, this position clearly advocates medical paternalism in some (if not most) instances of treatment-refusal by nondying patients. The physician's duty to care, which generally encompasses a duty to prolong life where possible, is not founded upon the patient's wishes per se; such "subjective" wishes do not have "the power to make medical interventions right or wrong."[28] The physician should be guided primarily by "objective medical determination" of the patient's physiological needs. Furthermore, as James Childress has pointed out, Ramsey's linkage of agent-care with medical indications could lead physicians to protect their own moral integrity by forcing life-prolonging treatments on patients whose refusals they disagree with, rather than simply withdrawing from the case on conscientious grounds ([7], p. 182). In the case of Elizabeth Bouvia, for example (see Chapter 1), Ramsey's position suggests not only that she has a covenantal obligation to accept nourishment and other life-prolonging treatment (despite her paralysis and painful arthritis), but also that her physicians and other care-givers have independent duties of "agent-care" not to "abandon" her – i.e., positively, to sustain her nondying condition with all medically indicated treatments.

We have seen in this discussion that there are inferential ambiguities in Ramsey's seeming approval of "dying well enough" coupled with his condemnation of choosing death. And we are left with the question of what exactly he means in affirming the "relative right to refuse treatment": *to what* is it relative, other than the patient's 'objective' medical status (i.e., 'nondying' or 'dying')? Let us conclude this section, though, by examining further two presumptions at the very foundation of his moral position: the logical entailments of a broad 'right to refuse treatment' and the moral entailments of his 'gift' and 'trust' metaphors for life itself.

First, consider Ramsey's syllogistic assertion:

If the claim were verified that an individual has a right to arbitrary self-determination in the matter of life and death, and if he then chooses to live, [then] there would be a duty upon others to protect his life; and, equally, if he chooses to die, there would be a duty upon others to assist his dying ([41], p. 158).

Ramsey holds it as true beyond argument that nobody has a *right* to another's assistance in his death – which is one reason why we have laws against assisted suicide (a matter very much under review in several states as I write this). And he argues backward from this truism to rebut any assumption of a "right to arbitrary self-determination" in personal life-or-death decisions on the grounds that a 'right to die' would necessarily entail a correlative duty of assistance by others. But is this a reasonable statement of the matter? It would seem, in fact, that Ramsey is conflating the notions of *positive* and *negative* rights and obligations[29] in a way that is neither necessary nor at all convincing.

Take, first, the case of an individual who choses to *live*. Surely we would submit to the proposition that anyone's decision (and claim) to remain living implies a duty on the part of others not to actively deny him life – in philosophical terms, a basic duty of non-maleficence. (Of course, historically we have not considered this duty to be *absolute*, as any perusal of just-war theories and arguments for capital punishment will attest.) More importantly, however, the duty not to deny another's life is a *negative* duty – a duty to *abstain* from doing something life-threatening to another. Now, if we decide that an individual's claim (or 'right') to stay alive also implies a separate, *positive* duty of assistance on the part of others (such as a moral obligation to provide health care),[30] we can (and do) derive that duty from moral sources *other than* the individual's claim not to be killed. Ramsey derives it, of course, from a more general duty of agent-care based upon covenant-fidelity, centered upon meeting neighbors' needs, and from his particular interpretation of the 'sanctity' of life. The point to be noted here, though, is that it is not logically necessary (in our history of reflection upon such matters, at least) to derive a positive duty of others' assistance solely from one's claim to be *allowed* to live.

So, why should one's wish *not* to remain alive logically entail anything like a positive duty of assistance from others? Remember that the context of Ramsey's argument is the patient's 'right to refuse treatment.' What possible meaning can the 'right to die' have in this context other than as a 'right to be left alone' (in terms of treatment)? A *positive* 'right to die' (with assistance) does not follow from a *negative* right to others' abstentions or forbearances; nor does it necessarily follow from any established positive right to assistance in staying alive. Ramsey's passion is really directed against those advocates of 'beneficent euthanasia' who assume the same fallacious logical sequence he does. Their approach is to derive a duty of (voluntary) euthanasic assistance from a particular interpretation of beneficence or 'mercy' (as a general moral obligation), then to insert it into the syllogistic sequence so as to imply a correlative, positive right on the part of those patients who desire such assistance. But these euthanasia advocates are thereby establishing *on other grounds* a claim which goes far beyond anything logically implied by a patient's right to refuse treatment.

Now, Ramsey's argument here is an example of a type of argument he frequently employs in *Ethics at the Edges* (and elsewhere), commonly called a 'wedge' or 'slippery slope' argument. The particular version he employs most often (as here) is sometimes called 'the hammer behind the wedge.' It focuses upon the process of moral reasoning about acts or rules and is concerned that we draw moral boundaries in such a way that our moral justifications of some actions do not logically entail extension to other, 'similar' actions we consider morally reprehensible (due to the moral and legal principle of universalizability: treat similar cases in a similar way).[31] In this instance, Ramsey is fearful that a right to assisted death *is* being (or will be) derived logically from an individual's right of self-determination (just as he has demonstrated). So he draws the moral boundary on the negative side of recognizing that right, in its fullest sense, at all.

But if the preceding critique of his argument is correct, and if we also accept a prima facie duty to respect patient autonomy as an expression of human "freedom and dignity," then we may well argue that Ramsey has drawn the boundary in the wrong place and has thereby overridden a basic moral principle – i.e., personal autonomy – without clear moral justification. Why not be satisfied to argue (as Ramsey *does* argue elsewhere) that any agent's negative obligations of care (e.g., 'refrain from killing') are morally prior to and stronger than positive obligations of 'mercy' (as individual interpretations of beneficence), and thus that the latter cannot support a positive duty *or* correlative right of assisted death? Ramsey would, after all, have plenty of clear examples for illustrating the discontinuity of positive and negative rights/duties (e.g., the negative right of free speech does not entail another's obligation to publish one's work, the negative right to own property does not entail another's duty to provide it, etc.). In short, the logical pile-driver Ramsey sees behind this 'wedge' is perhaps no more formidable than a tack-hammer – and is as easily arrested.

But, of course, Ramsey's agenda is broader than this not-so-logical threat of euthanasia-on-demand. He has other reasons for limiting any "right to arbitrary self-determination in the matter of life and death." So let us examine, as a final focus of this section, his understanding of the moral warrants implied in his religious metaphors of 'gift' and 'trust.'

Both metaphors are engaged specifically to illustrate not the 'sacredness' of human life in general, but rather one's particular relations to his/her own physical being and to God. And both metaphors can surely be said to have biblical foundations. The Genesis creation-stories describe God's gifts to Adam of both life and a name; many of Jesus's parables develop the notion of stewardship of what one has been given in trust; and so on. These and other scriptural expressions have given rise to a long tradition in Christianity of viewing our mortal lives as divine beneficences for which we should be grateful, and as personal responsibilities rather than corporeal chattels.

But even our confessions of gratitude for life's gift, and our responsibility for its stewardship, do not yet answer all questions of moral interpretation for those metaphors. What, for instance, are the *limits* of gratitude and trusteeship? Ramsey draws the conceptual line between choosing to live until one is medically 'dying,' on the one hand, and "choosing death" on the other. The latter choice signals "defeat" of God's gift-giving; it also "evidences a denial that God is trustworthy, or at least some doubt that he knew what he was doing when he called us by our own proper names and trusted us with life" ([41], p. 147). In the context of incurable patients' treatment-refusals, however, neither the exact onset of 'dying' nor the patient's singular will-to-die can be so clearly ascertained (even by the patient himself/herself, in many instances). Moreover, the central question here is not simply *whether* we will be stewards of our lives, but, more specifically, *what* choices for life-extending technology are required by our stewardship. And Ramsey's own view of the relationship between what is medically possible and what is morally required seems to have shifted over time. *The Patient as Person* referred to "medical progress" as a process of "constantly creating more and more extraordinary means that need not be used and perhaps ought not to be chosen [by incurable, nondying patients]" ([32], p. 141). *Ethics at the Edges of Life* hails these fruits of medical progress as "surely medically indicated and desirable" ([41], p. 156). Ramsey still maintains that stewardship does not entail 'vitalism,' in the sense of requiring life's prolongation no-matter-what. And his continued insistence upon a policy of at least seriously considering incurable patients' own treatment preferences certainly implies a flexibility of some degree. But his specific examples of genuinely 'optional' treatments are, in his later writings, narrowed to those that are medically nonbeneficial (in contrast to those that are personally burdensome).[32] So perhaps there is some truth in John Connery's suggestion that Ramsey is "canonizing medical indications."[33] At least he appears to be advocating a duty to preserve the gift of one's life until it becomes medically clear that the Giver will soon be taking it back.

We may yet ask, though, whether Ramsey's interpretive use of 'gift' and 'trust' as metaphors does full justice to the moral meaning of those terms. Metaphors generally function to clarify a particular idea or relationship by describing it as some other idea or relationship with which we are experientially familiar.[34] And perhaps Ramsey's metaphorical use of these notions tends to obscure some features we commonly associate with them. Do we, for instance, commonly consider a gift – even a gift-in-trust[35] – to be an irrevocable responsibility? Surely some entrusted gifts can become real *burdens*, at least to their particular trustees; and to return such a gift before return is requested (or demanded) is not flatly to "throw the gift back in the face of the giver." Nor is it to "defeat his gift-giving." In short, we *do* recognize morally valid reasons for returning an entrusted gift other than the giver's own express reclamation of it.[36] This is not to deny the appropriateness of characterizing *some* gift-rejections (and, by metaphorical application, some deliberate choices for death) as examples of ingratitude. It is simply to affirm that our experiences of gift-receiving and gift-returning offer moral explanations for the latter action other than ingratitude.[37]

In other words, the modest point being made here is that Ramsey's particular inferences about the "unfaithfulness" of choosing death, drawn ostensibly from reflection upon biblically (and experientially) supplied metaphors, are not the *only* reasonable inferences which may be drawn from those metaphors (or even from broader biblical testimony on the matter).[38] The reflections offered here, then, are not intended to – and cannot – confute Ramsey's claims. They are instead intended to suggest that perhaps his rhetorical arguments overextend his evidences for them.

Now, these critiques of Ramsey's supporting arguments have perhaps moved our discussion away from the concrete detail of covenant-obligation toward the sick and dying. Suffice it to say, though, that Ramsey's presentation leaves us with some significant and unresolved tensions among his various requirements of covenant-fidelity, requirements which include: the physician's duty to do what is 'medically indicated' in preserving life; his/her duty also to respect patients' own autonomous valuations of continued treatments; our (social) acceptance of those rules of practice which will most effectively deter assisted suicide and voluntary (or involuntary) euthanasia (as both are, in Ramsey's view, faithfulness-eroding practices); and the patient's obligation to maintain his/her own physical being as befits a divinely-entrusted beneficence. It does seem safe to conclude, however, that Ramsey's interpretation and 'weighting' of these requirements tends to mandate any and all treatments which are not useless – even at the expense of a given patient's 'right' of self-determination.

5. COVENANT-LOYALTY IN PEDIATRIC RESEARCH

Among the 'exceptionless' moral rules which follow from Ramsey's notion of covenant-fidelity is the requirement that all human subjects of medical experimentation give a voluntary, informed consent to their participation. Indeed, the principle of an informed consent is "the cardinal *canon of loyalty* joining men together in medical practice and investigation." In this requirement "faithfulness among men – the faithfulness that is normative for all the covenants or moral bonds of life with life – gains specification for the primary relations peculiar to medical practice" ([32], p. 5).

What can be said, then, of potential research subjects who are incapable of offering an informed consent for themselves – i.e., children and incompetent adults? Ramsey's answer is clear and unmistakable: persons who cannot give a mature, competent, and informed consent should *never* be made subjects of medical experimentation *unless* there are reasonable grounds for believing that participation promises medical benefit *for that patient-subject*. This answer is really two separate answers. First, it rejects outright any involvement of children (or incompetent adults) in nontherapeutic experimentation, regardless of the degree (or absence) of subject-risk involved or of the potential benefits to others. And, second, it allows for 'proxy' or surrogate consents in cases where experimental treatment may be of therapeutic benefit for the consent-less individual.

To treat Ramsey's latter answer first (and narrowing its focus to children), he is arguing that the covenant-requirement of informed consent may be stretched to include proxy consent by parents, but only on the basis of the child's own medical *needs*. "To consent in place of a child means to consent *in his behalf medically*, i.e., for medical reasons and possible benefit to him." This is the only sort of consent which falls within the nature and meaning of "the responsibilities of parenthood as a covenant among the generations of men" ([32], pp. 26, 39). It is also the only sort of consent which, in Ramsey's view, can be construed reasonably as what the child *would* give if (s)he could. As for the epistemological basis of such a construal, he cites his version of "a natural law conception of the human good," which, as we have seen, involves "an empirical comprehension of the goods to which human life naturally or observably directs itself" ([37], p. 22). Now, this looks at first very much like McCormick's order of human goods derived from "examining man's basic tendencies" as well. But Ramsey insists that McCormick has failed to distinguish between natural human inclinations *simpliciter* and natural human inclinations *in childhood*, and that the good to which childhood inclines is simply the preservation of life and a healthy life and growth. Thus, childhood interests and parental responsibilities converge in consenting only to those medical procedures aimed explicitly at somehow promoting the child's health and nurture.

Ramsey does point out, however, that experimentation may be construed sometimes as promoting the child's own good even if it is not immediately curative or palliative. He defends, for example, Jonas Salk's extensive trials of polio vaccine on large populations of healthy children. Because each of the children involved was already at risk of contracting polio if exposed to it, their parents were balancing on their behalf the risks of the trial against the benefits of acquired immunity *for the individual child-subject*. Thus, Ramsey is willing to amend the rule, "Never subject children to the unknown possible hazards of medical investigations having no relation to their own treatment," to include the qualification, ". . . except in epidemic conditions" ([32], p. 15).

But does this nevertheless mean – contra McCormick – that the child's good can never also be construed so as to include the health and nurture of *other* children, children who may be greatly benefited by the child's nontherapeutic research participation? In Ramsey's estimation, it means exactly that.

> To attempt to consent for a child to be made an experimental subject [in nontherapeutic research] is to treat a child as not a child. It is to treat him as if he were an adult person who has consented to become a joint adventurer in the common cause of medical research. If the grounds for this are alleged to be the presumptive or implied consent of the child, that must simply be characterized as a violent and false presumption ([32], p. 14).

Like McCormick, Ramsey is arguing that any morally valid proxy consent for a child must be, in essence, a 'substituted judgement' – a well-founded presumption of what the child *would* choose if (s)he were capable of doing so. Unlike McCormick, however, Ramsey rejects any further presumption of what the child *should* choose, if that presumption involves a child's obligation to further anyone else's interests. What is clearly supposed in this view is that a young child would (and by natural inclination *should*) choose the childhood good of self-preservation and healthful growth. But he/she is not yet a mature, socialized individual, and thus would have no reason for choosing to bear "obligations that hitherto have been supposed to be only electable by persons in the adult world" ([37], p. 23). The key terms here are "adult" and "electable." Not only would proxy consent for nontherapeutic research be treating a child as an adult; it would also be treating a child as an adult who had chosen the moral *option* of benefiting others.

This is an important point, for it highlights a critical difference in perspective between Ramsey and McCormick about what is going on, morally, in the very enterprise of medical experimentation. McCormick advocates fully voluntary participation in human experimentation as the best possible moral arrangement. But he also derives a minimal duty of social justice that we all (including children) share and that obliges us to be willing to accept minimal or negligible burdens (i.e., research risks) in order to produce benefits for us all. As he puts it, "[i]f we really expect to, want to, and demand to enjoy the fruits of medical progress, we should be willing to bear our share in the development of this progress" ([18], p. 2179). While this claim is conditional rather than categorical, McCormick clearly assumes the 'good' of medical progress per se to be not only morally desirable but in some sense morally obligatory (at least where the burdens or risks are minimal). It is for this reason that he rejects the language of 'charitable works' and insists instead upon referring to participation in minimal-risk research as a duty of *justice*, of "one's personal bearing of his share of the burden."

In contrast, Ramsey views this interpretation as fundamentally mistaken. He believes that the so-called "research imperative" – the zeal of researchers to discover and test new treatments and cures – does have moral meaning, but only as an expression of our positive duties to *benefit* others, to "do good." These duties are not as stringent as our negative duties to "avoid evil": "In general, one does not have the same duty to help people as to refrain from injuring them" ([39], p. 41). The most stringent moral duty in medical research, as in clinical practice, is summarized in the Hippocratic dictum, *primum non nocere* ("above all, do no harm"). Neither the community's general duty to benefit the sick (present and future) through nontherapeutic research, nor any individual's duty to benefit his peers, can be presumed to be more compelling than our primary duty to avoid harming research subjects. And even when the potential research risks in question are 'minimal' or 'negligible,' we are "still speaking of doing calculable harm to bring aid." So we cannot assume anything like a *duty* of justice on the part of unconsenting potential subjects of nontherapeutic research. Of course, those who *can* consent and who choose to do so thereby become covenantal "partners" in the beneficent quest for medical advances; they voluntarily choose to accept research risks which they have no generalizable duty to bear. Ramsey's central point, though, is that research participation – and medical advancement in general – amounts to a morally *optional* undertaking. He agrees with Hans Jonas in insisting upon "the essentially gratutious nature of the whole enterprise of progress, as against the mandatory respect for invasion-proof selfhood" ([32], p. 109). In Ramsey's view, then, McCormick's rationalization of a presumptive minimal duty to participate amounts to "the enforcement of morals," or at least "the enforcement of minimum sociality" ([39], p. 40).

Given the tenets of Ramsey's position considered thus far – that our primary medical duty is to avoid harm and that the good young children seek is their own healthy development (only) – one might still argue that perhaps there are research protocols to which a child *would not object*, even if (s)he is as yet unable to offer an informed consent. Imagine, for example, a protocol in which children are fed a diet of normal, healthful foods that have been carefully measured and prepared; then the childrens' urine is collected at certain intervals and assayed to determine relative concentrations of excretory byproducts. There is no particular therapeutic benefit for the children-subjects in all of this. Suppose, further, that the data obtained will be of great benefit in controlling the diets of children undergoing antibiotic treatment for a relatively rare bladder infection (and that data obtained from assays of adult urine cannot be correlated accurately with pediatric excretory function). In such a scenario, the child-subject's own good of healthy development would be neither threatened nor therapeutically advanced, nor would the researchers be exposing normal children to any measurable risk of harm. So, it would seem quite reasonable to some, then, to assume that the child-subject would not *object* to his parent's proxy consent for his participation.

But Ramsey would reject this argument as well. In his view, even (nontherapeutic) research that does not add to the "ordinary risks of childhood" should nevertheless not involve unconsenting children as subjects. For also at issue is "the wrong of making a human being an 'object' and using him in trials not in his behalf as a subject" ([32], p. 36). On this point Ramsey appeals to Immanuel Kant's famous 'categorical imperative' which (in Kant's second formulation of it) forbids using any human person only as a *means* to one's own, or anybody else's, ends. While Kant grounded this imperative in his assumption that humanity, in oneself or in others, is the source of all rational moral self-legislation, Ramsey insists that the same requirement follows from our recognition of "the wholeness of God's care for the least and the littlest ones and their preciousness to Him" ([37], p. 30, n. 19). And in his view of the matter at hand, experimentation "possibly or even remotely connected" with a child-subject's own treatment is "the *outer limit* of procedures that treat a child-patient as an 'end *also*' and never as a 'means *only*'" ([37], p. 26). Because a child cannot consent to, and adopt as his own, the ends or goals of nontherapeutic research, he cannot truly become a *subject* of that research. Proxy consent would make him a mere *object* of research – a 'means' to someone else's investigational ends.

Ramsey finds further support for this moral argument in the Anglo-American legal tradition. Under the law, he tells us, one can claim injury (through negligence or battery, e.g.) if some harmful invasion of his body has been commenced without his consent. He can also claim the injury of "unconsented touching" – a coercion or harmless offense by the will of another, which still counts as an assault even if no harm is done.[39] Applied to the situation of children in nontherapeutic research, then, "they could be *harmfully* used, or they could simply be *used* with no harm"; but in either case they would be wronged ([32], p. 37). And a policy of allowing such research would deprive children of the protections of law in both respects. It would amount, both morally and legally, to "a sanitized form of barbarism" ([32], p. 12).

For all these reasons (and more) Ramsey insists we should hold to the rule of informed consent as an exceptionless canon of medical morality, which means that we should never allow the participation of children in nontherapeutic experimentation.

Moreover, while these primary arguments appeal to what Ramsey calls "faithfulness claims," he also offers a (familiar) consequence-oriented argument for disallowing any exceptions of informed consent as a rule of practice. For, medical progress is not the only attractive result of experimentation; it is also the case that the researcher "rises to the top" in medicine through the significance and success of his work. Therefore,

... [t]he likelihood that a researcher would make a mistake in departing from a generally valuable rule of medical practice [the rule of informed consent] because he is biased toward the research benefits of permitting an 'exception' is exceedingly great. In such a seriously important moral matter, this should be enough to rebut a policy of being open to future possible exceptions to this canon of medical ethics . . .

. . . If every doer loves his deed more than it ought to be loved, so every researcher his research – and, of course, its promise of future benefits for mankind . . . To assume otherwise would be to assume an equally serene rationality on the part of men in all moral matters. It would be to assume that a man is as able to sustain good moral judgement and to make a proper choice with a strong interest in results obtainable by violating the requirements of an informed consent as he would be if he had no such interest ([32], pp. 9–10).

This secondary and supportive argument exemplifies another form of the 'wedge' or 'slippery slope' argument. But, unlike the logical 'hammer behind the wedge' argument (described above in Section 4), the present form, sometimes called 'what the wedge is driven into,' is not concerned with logical extensions of our exception-making but rather with the erosion of our commitment to moral rules as a consequence of making more and more exceptions to them. The particular fear expressed here is that researchers will begin to find many good reasons for not treating patient-subjects as autonomous 'ends' in themselves. And the practice of requiring voluntary, informed consent will be eroded if we allow any exceptions whatever.

In summary, then, we have seen that Ramsey offers both fidelity-claims and consequentialist reasons for rejecting any proxy consent for the involvement of children in nontherapeutic research. Before concluding this section, however, we should also take note of his own description of the most plausible *alternative* to his position. In a paper presented at the 1973 Conference on Biological Revolution/Theological Impact [34], Ramsey outlined what he considers the best moral case for a view which was already prevalent within the medical research community itself – namely, that proxy consent for children in nontherapeutic research may be valid in some cases (where experimental risks are minimal and prospective benefits for other children are great). He notes a general social move toward the language of 'rights' of future generations, and of our correlative obligations to provide medical benefits for them – as against the inviolable 'rights' of current research subjects. And he suggests that if we really consider the former rights/obligations to be equally weighty with the latter (as Ramsey himself does not), then perhaps the model of moral life which presents itself is one of possibly irreducible conflict of principles – a model of 'tragic choices' which offers "no rational or principled way to decide or harmonize these claims" and which requires that we choose the lesser apparent evil. Ramsey refers to this as a "peculiarly Protestant" understanding of moral life, one which stresses our fallen nature as a source of moral ambiguity rather than clear moral guidance and which therefore emphasizes the evilness of either choice in such decisions. He adverts to Michael Walzer's well-known discussion of "the problem of dirty hands" in political decision-making (in which a political leader advances the 'common good' by knowingly 'doing wrong' and bearing the guilt and responsibility for it) as an illustration of this sort of quandary-ethics. And he suggests that perhaps this view would recognize some "borderline situations" in nontherapeutic experimentation where moral agents are under the necessity of doing wrong [by using unconsenting subjects] for the public good. Under such circumstances, we would properly expect the responsible moral agents to realize the weight of evil in their choices. So, Ramsey remarks in very "Protestant" tones, "[i]t is by their feelings of moral suffering and guilt that we know the physician worthy (if anyone is) to experiment on children or others incapable of consenting in their own right" ([34], p. 62). Moreover, we would also choose to compromise, or limit the extent of our wrongdoing, by deeming the selection of nonconsenting children a "class action," thus limiting their experimental use to research aimed solely at solving medical problems of children as a class of persons.

This, then, comprises the most powerful argument Ramsey believes available to his rhetorical opponents. It has the virtue of offering an understanding of "how to do research with children without loosening moral bonds or weakening moral claims in a broken and fallen world" ([37], p. 21). But he is quick to remind us that it also has many vices. The most foundational one is that the moral vision it represents "takes the ethic of ambiguity to be especially revelatory of the nature and dilemmas of moral decision in general" ([34], p. 64). As a result, it seeks to make a virtue of its own inability to resolve moral conflicts through the exercise of moral reason. And, of course, it assumes in this case a parity or commensurability of competing moral claims which Ramsey is not inclined to accept. (In particular, he sees a great need for us to de-escalate our current "imperatives of research" if we are to assess correctly the morality of any experiment "in its inception.")

While it is quite clear that Ramsey considers this second, "peculiarly Protestant" position vastly inferior to his original one, what is not so clear is his *purpose* in constructing and presenting the second argument at all – especially since he has done so with such clarity and thoughtfulness. Some commentators have suggested that it reflects Ramsey's own discomfort with the bleak consequences (for pediatric medicine) of his former, absolutistic position. In this view, Ramsey is pictured as 'yielding' some of his original high moral ground to a more intuitively acceptable alternative (see, e.g., [19]).

Another possibility is that the alternative position is merely a heuristic device by which Ramsey hopes to convince us of the soundness and inescapability of his former conclusions; his own later references to this "Protestant" proposal as a "thought experiment" and as an argument presented "hypothetically" tend to offer some credence to this interpretation ([37], p. 21; [38], p. 212). Nevertheless, his latest writings on the subject continue to defend it as preferable to various other moral options (save his own absolutist position). He has insisted, for example, that *both* of his proposed solutions "are superior to McCormick's" ([37], p. 21).

There is, however, yet a third possible light in which we might view Ramsey's 'plan B.' We have seen at several points that one of his central concerns is for the *ethos* of our modern culture; he worries that we are moving toward moral justification of what is (for him) morally unjustifiable. Now, note that what both of his 'positions' on pediatric research have in common is that neither of them *justifies* nontherapeutic experimentation with children. One position condemns it outright; the other suggests that it may be in some cases a necessary, though guilt-producing, *evil*. Further, Ramsey was formulating both arguments at a time when the current of opinion in the research, bioethical, and public policy communities was moving toward justification of at least some minimal-risk nontherapeutic research involving children. Perhaps, then, his latter position represents an attempt at moral 'damage control' with respect to the foundations of public policy. In other words, perhaps he was offering us a way of understanding that what we are not willing to forbid (out of concern for sick children to come) is not thereby *right* by default. For, while this "Protestant" proposal admits the possibility of 'borderline' experimentation situations in which it may be tragically necessary for the researcher to accept "dirty hands" in order to benefit future sick children, it nonetheless emphasizes the wrongness of such actions along with their perceived necessity. And in this way it retains some of the morally restraining force of Ramsey's original position as a presumptive standard.

Moreover, Ramsey freely affirms that "among wrong actions, some are wronger than others." And he rarely hesitates to point out *which* actions and reasons for acting are more and less wrong. For instance, he is convinced of the wrongness of artificial insemination by donor (AID) because it rends asunder the God-given unity of sexual love and procreation; but he concedes that *if* AID is to be allowed by law, then it would be a "better wrong" morally to practice it with a view toward giving the potential child a "better [healthier] genetic inheritance" than simply to produce a child who looks as much like the legal parents as possible ([31], esp. Chapter 1). Likewise, it is a "better wrong" to conduct pediatric research with full appreciation of its violations of covenant-fidelity (and a restraining sense of one's wrongdoing) than to proceed under the assumption that prospective benefits for future children really outweigh our immediate covenantal obligations to present research subjects.

Pulling these reflections together, one might argue that Ramsey's practical aim in sketching a "Protestant" alternative to his own position was simply (in terminology familiar to Calvinists and Lutherans) the "restraint of sin" – in this case, the restraint of any shift in our social ethos toward purely consequentialist *justification* of present covenant-violations. It is perhaps instructive to recall here that in *Basic Christian Ethics* Ramsey emphasized restraint of sin as the primary concern of "Christian love in search of a social policy." And surely his tendency to differentiate and define greater and lesser moral 'sins' can be read as an ongoing expression of that concern in his own exhortations about social practices. If this admittedly speculative view of Ramsey's purpose is correct, then he is certainly carrying forward here a major emphasis of Reformation social thought, since both Luther and Calvin considered the restraint of sin to be one of the primary 'uses' of the divine moral law. And in that sense, at least, Ramsey may have had historically "Protestant" reasons for offering his "peculiarly Protestant" proposal.

* * *

The reader is certainly aware by now that Ramsey's theological-ethical perspective incorporates a rich and wide-ranging amalgam of both faith-centered and experientially-based claims. His particular points of emphasis have shifted somewhat over the years, largely in order to sharpen his defenses of his "mixed agapism" against the counter-claims of various other ethical approaches – Catholic natural law theory, utilitarianism, and fideistic intuitionism, to name but a few. What has never changed, however, is his insistence upon *agape*, expressed through the demands of "covenant fidelity," as the central norm for all human attitudes and behaviors. God's covenant-faithfulness toward each of us provides the model for our loyalties to each other in all the 'orders' of our created existence; God's willingness to be bound by his covenant-promises provides the model for our willingness to accept love-embodying rules of practice (and our experience of the need for consistency and continuity in moral life provides a congruent stimulus).

Perhaps the most controversial aspect of Ramsey's moral theory is his derivation of exceptionless moral rules. He claims to have proven the logical possibility of such rules, and he is certainly not shy about identifying and applying them in the contexts of medical treatment and research! Indeed, his zeal in doing so has led to the charge that his theory evidences a "creeping legalism."[40] But at least we can probably all agree that Ramsey is one of contemporary Christian ethics' most militant defenders against "creeping exceptionism."

This chapter has also highlighted some of the profound differences between Ramsey's theological ethics and Richard McCormick's – e.g., their divergent theologies of death, their different understandings of 'natural law', their methodological differences concerning the role of ends and consequences in moral decision making, and so on. Before proceeding further in our study, however, we should note that their disparate methods share substantial common ground. Both moralists have adumbrated theories applicable to choosing and judging particular actions and practices. Both theories derive concrete norms of behavior, be they based upon value-realization or covenantal obligation. In short, both have had much to say about *what* we should *do* (or not do), either in terms of the goods we should seek or the obligations we should meet. So, McCormick and Ramsey are at least "within shouting distance" methodologically, as Lisa Cahill has so aptly put it [5].

Yet act-analysis, and justification of acts and practices, does not exhaust the range of either ancient or contemporary moral reflection. There are, indeed, theologians and moral philosophers who claim that the primary focus of any ethics should be the qualities, attitudes or perspectives of moral agents themselves rather than the rightness/wrongness of their deeds per se or the goodness of their achieved ends or consequences. And the next chapter of this study will explore the work of a contemporary Christian moralist who exemplifies that focus upon agent-morality: Stanley Hauerwas.

NOTES

[1] [23], p. 149. Some have argued that Ramsey misunderstands Thomas's notion of charity, which involves love of the neighbor "for his own sake." See, e.g., [4], esp. p. 218, n. 2.

[2] [23], p. 339. This assertion lays the groundwork for Ramsey's later resolution of the faith/reason dialectic in terms of "love transforming natural justice."

[3] Even in the Christian's search for a social policy, "the final word must place the accent again on freedom, freedom even from the social policies Christian love may have found in times past" ([23], p. 351).

[4] [25], p. 28f. In the "Afterword" of *Christian Ethics and the Sit-In* Ramsey offers "faith effective through in-principled love" and "Christ transforming natural justice" as synonymous notions (pp. 124–28).

[5] [25], p. 48. Earlier, in *Basic Christian Ethics*, Ramsey had also cited "restraint of sin" as the primary concern of Christian ethics in its search for appropriate social policies.

[6] [25], p. 48f. Ramsey does propose a sort of theory of justified revolution in *The Just War*, at least where order stands ready to replace the older order, where revolution is the last resort, and where all other means of achieving a more just order have been tried first (see [30], esp. pp. 458–64, 528).

[7] Because Ramsey's topical writings in medical ethics will be our central concern here, his very influential writings in just war theory will receive little attention. It is certainly worth noting here, however, that his interpretation of just war doctrine is also profoundly *love*-dominant. While the tradition has appealed explicitly to notions of natural justice and natural right in developing doctrine, the overall thrust of it was originally, in Ramsey's view, concern for the present needs of the neighbor. Love for the neighbor sometimes requires force for the protection of the innocent; it also requires norms for the limitation of force – i.e., the principle of non-combatant immunity (and, secondarily, the principle of proportionality in the means of warfare). Such norms provide further examples of love 'transforming' natural justice. (See, e.g., [26], pp. xviii–xxi, 49, 190–91, 305–6; and [30], Chapters 6 and 7.)

[8] Lisa Cahill points out that, in addition to the congruence of moral norms derived from natural and revealed "covenants," Ramsey's topical writings manifest two other reasons for his expectation of a "covergence" between religious and humanistic moral judgements: (1) the influence and affirmation of Christian values in Western culture; and (2) the suggestion that God's redemptive covenant is itself all-inclusive (see [5], pp. 398–400).

[9] William F. May, for example, offers a more reciprocal model of medical relationships in *The Physician's Covenant* [20].

[10] [23], p. 77. His most extensive arguments – particularly against the relativism he sees in

the views of John A.T. Robinson, Paul Lehmann, and Joseph Fletcher – are collected in *Deeds and Rules in Christian Ethics* [29].

[11] Ramsey's distinction between "summary rules" and "rules of practices" is drawn from John Rawls' article, "Two Concepts of Rules" [44].

[12] See Section 2 of Chapter 2 for McCormick's discussion of the same case.

[13] [22], p. 87f. Of course, those who remain unconvinced by this particular interpretation may be led to ask, What sorts of *limits* are there to Ramsey's rather creative redefinitions of rules in order to find implicit meanings which may be made explicit in the prism of this case? After all, Mrs. Bergmeier's act-justification, as Ramsey presents it, seems to hinge upon the lovingness of the particular *consequence* she *hopes* to bring about by her deed, and not any loving quality in the deed itself, even if she (and we) are willing to say it would be 'right' in all other relevantly similar cases.

[14] [22], pp. 109, 114. Ramsey also insists that the defender of exceptionless rules is not simply giving top priority to "collective or social values" at the *expense* of openness to exceptions which may give priority to the neighbor's good in the situation. Rather, he is seeking to "build a floor under the individual fellow man by minimum faithfulness-rules or canons of loyalty to him that are unexceptionable, while it is the proponent of future possible exceptions who may be placing societal and gross consequence-values uppermost" (p. 133).

[15] [22], pp. 127–33. He also cites, in his argument for exceptionless rules of practice, the moral proscriptions of premarital sex (although he allows that the covenantal relationship of "marriage" may exist pre-ceremonially) and of punishing a man for something of which one knows him to be innocent (116f., 108). One of Ramsey's critics, Donald Evans, has suggested that Ramsey makes too absolute a claim for exceptionless moral rules. Evans agrees that the criterion of universalizability bans *singular* justifiable exceptions, and that exceptionless moral rules are *logically* possible. But he holds the real issue to be "*Should* there be such exceptionless rules?" And he gives counter-examples to some of Ramsey's examples in order to show that we should instead accept some rules as "*virtually* exceptionless" only. This insistence, Evans writes, "is a check on creeping legalism" ([10], pp. 160–96). See also Gene Outka's discussion in [21].

[16] An important caveat must be entered here. The explication of Ramsey's argument presented in this section has emphasized his rule-strengthening claims; but the "freedom of *agape*" and the necessity of agential *prudence* (in subsuming cases) are also very much alive and in dialectical evidence in his argument. Indeed, Ramsey himself has cited, as a "correct summary" of his argumentative accomplishment in "The Case of the Curious Exception," Paul Camenisch's conclusion about that article: ". . . Ramsey's impressive argumentation on behalf of exceptionless principles and rules has resulted in giving us the *possibility* of *negative* rules and principles which require a *continuing interpretation* to discern what they forbid, are to be held to as exceptionless only in the *absence* of love-violating counter-instances, and are prohibited by the inviolable rights of prudence from making pronouncements in individual cases" ([6], p. 84).

[17] [35], p. 51. Ramsey's specifically theological reflections on death center around the Pauline correlation of sin and death. Sin is seen to be the 'cause' of death, and the existential anxiety introduced in us by the fact of death produces sin in turn. 'Redemption' in this view means our release from the power of sin and death; for, "perfect love casts out any fear of loss of life" (see [27]). Significantly, though, he focuses solely upon the existential import of our redemption from dread and sin. Death may be 'conquered' in the eyes of faith, but the terrible event of death is not transformed to any positive conclusion of life. Ramsey does not offer any particular interpretation of post-death resurrection destiny, and he does explicitly reject the identification of "eternal life" with "immortality of the soul." So, any Ramseyan theology of "eternal life" is unclear, at best, beyond its liberating existential significance (see [4], Chapter 8).

[18] [32], pp. xii–xiii. Some critics have questioned whether Ramsey can (or does) consistently derive his version of a sanctity-of-life principle from his earlier explanations of *agape*. See, for example, Charles Harris, "Love as the Basic Moral Principle in Paul Ramsey's Ethics" [15].

[19] Ramsey himself would prefer that the courts not become, in effect, "state-wide institutional review boards" for treatment decisions – especially, no doubt, since he believes that the courts' *Quinlan*, *Saikewicz* and *Eichner* decisions were based on wrong reasons. But his basic stake in the procedural issue is really that of guaranteeing right choices, *"whoever decides."*

[20] [32], p. 161. Note Ramsey's descriptive *language* in referring to these two groups of dying patients – especially in contrast to McCormick's description of very similar patients. Ramsey condones some acts of complete treatment-withdrawal – and even euthanasia – because the patient "already is *beyond* our love and care" and "in impenetrable solitude." This denotes rather an acknowledgement of defeat and already-separation. McCormick, on the other hand, would justify treatment-withdrawal (but not euthanasia) for a patient whose life, due to conditions quite similar to those Ramsey describes, "can be said to have *achieved* its *potential*." Surely it would be difficult to avoid surmising that these two linguistic expressions of the same phenomenon are informed by *very different* attitudes about death!

[21] Ramsey cagily avoided making this descriptive statement explicitly, repeating instead over and over again that it "was the finding of both courts." Nevertheless, his discussion appears to assume its accuracy (see [41], pp. 268–72).

[22] [41], pp. 214–17. It should be noted that the very possibility of collapsing this distinction in any case involving a *child* is a striking and unusual departure for Ramsey – at least for the Ramsey of *Ethics at the Edges*. For, one of the points he makes repeatedly in that volume is that the moral killing/letting die distinction, to which we have traditionally held in adult care, is not applicable in infant care – that in fact, letting a defenseless baby die is morally equivalent to killing him. It is an immoral desertion of "one of God's little ones," regardless of the handicaps the little one may have.

[23] And Ramsey gives no indication of willingness to justify abortion of a fetus diagnosed with this disease prenatally.

[24] [45], cited by Ramsey in [41], pp. 180–81. Notice that this criterion, coupled with Ramsey's medical indications policy as already stated, comprise the essential features of mandated treatment (and exclusions) in the Child Abuse Amendments of 1984 (P.L. 98–457) cited in Chapter 1, above. Ramsey has expressed general satisfaction with that legislation's guidelines (in conversation with this writer), but he would have preferred that a stronger sanction be attached to the new law. Specifically, he would have preferred that the issue be addressed under tort law rather than constitutional law, since the threat of a lawsuit for financial damages would provide a more powerful deterrent to 'wrong' treatment decisions by parents and physicians.

[25] Lisa Cahill has argued that within a notion of agential (physician) responsibility, perhaps the exceptions (to the presumption for life-prolonging care) "might be allowed not by a tactic which avoids covenant responsibilities but by one which fulfills them." So her suggestion to Ramsey is that his possible allowance even of acts of euthanasia would be better presented as "the present *requirement* of our covenant fidelity" to the patient in some limited circumstances, rather than as an assumption of covenant-care's impossibility (see [3], pp. 470–76).

[26] In fact, the unqualified term "indicated" finds an enormous variety of applications in medical parlance. Quite a few physicians of my acquaintance use the phrase "X is indicated" to mean "I think X would be good for this patient" in a broadly evaluative sense. (A similarly omnivalent term in hospital nursing practice is "appropriate," which can indicate all sorts of judgments, ranging from the cognitive 'fit' of a patient's responses to verbal stimuli, to the perceived justifiability of a nurse's harsh response to his/her superior's orders, to the clinical usefulness of some new treatment mode for a given patient.)

[27] While these comments would appear to be aimed specifically at the professing Christian reader

or patient, Ramsey offers no such specification. Indeed, here he seems to assume a rather remarkable "covergence" between religious and humanistic moral judgements (see note 8, above).

[28] [41], p. 157. While arguing against 'external' conditions as improper patient-reasons for *refusing* treatment, Ramsey does point to such conditions as proper grounds for *overriding* such refusals. He approves, for instance, of court-ordered treatment for those who would "abandon children by trivial but suicidal refusals of treatment" (see [43], p. 133).

[29] See Joel Feinberg's discussion of positive and negative rights in his *Social Philosophy* [11].

[30] For an insightful collection of essays on "Rights to Health Care," see *The Journal of Medicine and Philosophy* 4/2 (June 1979).

[31] See James Childress, "Ethical Issues in Death and Dying" [7], for a discussion of Ramsey's wedge arguments. See also [41], pp. 306–07, fn.

[32] In this respect, it is interesting that Ramsey now insists that the older language of ordinary/extraordinary treatments always directed the attention of all involved to "*objective consideration of the patient's condition and of the armamentarium of medicine's remedies*," and that these considerations determined the moral rightness/wrongness of the patient's treatment refusals ([41], p. 157). This is certainly true up to a point; but the personal burdensomeness of treatment was also a key factor. We could hardly say, for example, that one's aversion to leaving home for treatment or submitting to disfiguring surgery would constitute "objective" considerations in Ramsey's use of the term. Yet they were acceptable justifications for refusing life-prolonging treatment in the tradition of Catholic moral theology.

[33] [8], p. 161. Connery's principal concern is Ramsey's strict exclusion of all quality-of-life considerations in proxy treatment decisions. My own contention is that Ramsey's zeal to avoid those considerations is also affecting his views on what sort of quality-of-life assessments competent incurables should be allowed to make for themselves.

[34] George Lakoff and Mark Johnson have offered insightful analyses of the interpretive and prescriptive power of commonplace metaphors in their *Metaphors We Live By* [17].

[35] To be consistent with Ramsey's application of these notions, we must consider them jointly (i.e., 'gifts-in-trust') as he does, since 'gift' alone carries connotations of full transfer of proprietary ownership, and 'trust' or 'stewardship' alone connotes a bilateral agreement in which responsibility for the entrusted property is willingly and explicitly accepted by the trustee. These connotations are among those Ramsey seeks to *avoid* highlighting!

[36] It is interesting to note that, unlike some religio-moral opponents of suicide who invoke the gift-of-life metaphor, Ramsey does not speak of "throwing the gift *away*"; he speaks instead of throwing it "back in the face of the giver." Thus, his metaphorical construct seems to recognize that this particular gift cannot be thrown *away from* this particular Giver! And my critique of his metaphorical use follows his lead in this regard by raising the question of when we think it appropriate to *return* a gift (rather than asking when it is appropriate to *destroy* or *throw away* a gift).

[37] For an excellent analysis of religious arguments against suicide based upon gift metaphors and analogies, see Margaret Pabst Battin, *Ethical Issues in Suicide* [2], esp. Chapter 1.

[38] These metaphors, and the broader biblical witness concerning 'choosing death,' will be considered further in Chapter 6.

[39] [32], p. 37. Interestingly, Ramsey somehow fails to mention this legal point in his discussion of treatment-refusals by competent patients!

[40] See note 15, above.

REFERENCES

1. Allen, J.L.: 1979, 'Paul Ramsey and His Respondents Since *The Patient as Person*', *Religious Studies Review* 5/2, 89–95.

2. Battin, M.P.: 1982, *Ethical Issues in Suicide*, Prentice-Hall, Englewood Cliffs, NJ.
3. Cahill, L.S.: 1975, 'Paul Ramsey: Covenant Fidelity in Medical Ethics', *Journal of Religion* 55 (October), 470–76.
4. Cahill, L.S.: 1976, 'Euthanasia: A Catholic and a Protestant Perspective', unpublished Ph.D. dissertation, University of Chicago.
5. Cahill, L.S.: 1979, 'Within Shouting Distance: Paul Ramsey and Richard McCormick on Method', *Journal of Medicine and Philosophy* 4/4, 398–417.
6. Camenisch, P.F.: 1974, 'Paul Ramsey's Task: Some Methodological Clarifications and Questions', in J.T. Johnson and D.H. Smith (eds.), *Love and Society: Essays in the Ethics of Paul Ramsey*, Scholar's Press, Missoula, Montana, pp. 67–89.
7. Childress, J.F.: 1978, 'Ethical Issues in Death and Dying', *Religious Studies Review* 4/3, 180–88.
8. Connery, J.R.: 1980, 'Prolonging Life: The Duty and Its Limits', *Lineacre Quarterly* 47/2, 151–65.
9. Curran, C.E.: 1973, *Politics, Medicine, and Christian Ethics: A Dialogue With Paul Ramsey*, Fortress Press, Philadelphia.
10. Evans, D.: 1980, *Faith, Authenticity, and Morality*, University of Toronto Press, Toronto.
11. Feinberg, J.: 1973, *Social Philosophy*, Prentice-Hall, Englewood Cliffs, NJ.
12. Frankena, W.: 1963, 'Love and Principle in Christian Ethics', in A. Plantinga (ed.), *Faith and Philosophy*, Prentice-Hall, Englewood Cliffs, NJ, pp. 203–25.
13. Frankena, W.: 1973, *Ethics*, 2nd ed., Prentice-Hall, Englewood Cliffs, NJ.
14. Goodman, E.: 1985, 'High Society Drama Now Private Horror', *The Daily Progress* (Charlottesville, VA), June 15, p. A4.
15. Harris, C.E., Jr.: 1976, 'Love as the Basic Moral Principle in Paul Ramsey's Ethics', *Journal of Religious Ethics* 4/2, 239–58.
16. Hoitenga, D.J., Jr.: 1970, 'Development of Paul Ramsey's Ethics', *Gordon Review* 11/5, 282–90.
17. Lakoff, G. and Johnson, M.: 1980, *Metaphors We Live By*, University of Chicago Press, Chicago.
18. McCormick, R.A.: 1976, 'Experimental Subjects: Who Should They Be?' *Journal of the American Medical Association* 235, 2197.
19. McCormick, R.A.: 1976, 'Experimentation in Children: Sharing in Sociality', *Hastings Center Report* 6/6, 41–46.
20. May, W.F.: 1983, *The Physician's Covenant: Images of the Healer in Medical Ethics*, Westminster Press, Philadelphia.
21. Outka, G.: 1984, 'The Protestant Tradition and Exceptionless Moral Norms', in *Moral Theology Today: Certitudes and Doubts*, The Pope John Center, St. Louis, MO, pp. 136–64.
22. Outka, G. and Ramsey, P. (eds.): 1968, *Norm and Context in Christian Ethics*, Charles Scribner's Sons, New York.
23. Ramsey, P.: 1950, *Basic Christian Ethics*, Charles Scribner's Sons, New York.
24. Ramsey, P.: 1960, 'Faith Effective Through In-Principled Love', *Christianity and Crisis* 20, 76–78.
25. Ramsey, P.: 1961, *Christian Ethics and the Sit-In*, Association Press, New York.
26. Ramsey, P.: 1961, *War and the Christian Conscience: How Shall Modern War Be Conducted Justly?*, Duke University Press, Durham, NC.
27. Ramsey, P.: 1962, 'Death's Duel', *Motive* 22/7, 2–5.
28. Ramsey, P.: 1962, *Nine Modern Moralists*, Prentice-Hall, Inglewood Cliffs, NJ.
29. Ramsey, P.: 1967, *Deeds and Rules in Christian Ethics*, Charles Scribner's Sons, New York.
30. Ramsey, P.: 1968, *The Just War: Force and Political Responsibility*, Charles Scribner's Sons, New York.

31. Ramsey, P.: 1970, *Fabricated Man: The Ethics of Genetic Control*, Yale University Press, New Haven.
32. Ramsey, P.: 1970, *The Patient as Person: Explorations in Medical Ethics*, Yale University Press, New Haven.
33. Ramsey, P.: 1971, 'The Ethics of a Cottage Industry in an Age of Community and Research Medicine', *New England Journal of Medicine* 284, 700–706.
34. Ramsey, P.: 1973, 'Medical Progress and Canons of Loyalty to Experimental Subjects', in *Proceedings of Conference on Biological Revolution/Theological Impact*, Institute for Theological Encounter with Science and Technology, St. Louis, MO, pp. 51–77.
35. Ramsey, P.: 1974, 'The Indignity of "Death with Dignity"', *Hastings Center Studies* 2/2, 47–62.
36. Ramsey, P.: 1974, 'Death's Pedagogy', *Commonweal* 100 (Sept. 20), 497–502.
37. Ramsey, P.: 1976, 'The Enforcement of Morals: Nontherapeutic Research on Children', *Hastings Center Report* 6/4, 21–30.
38. Ramsey, P.: 1976, 'Some Rejoinders', *Journal of Religious Ethics* 4/2, 185–237.
39. Ramsey, P.: 1977, 'Children as Research Subjects: A Reply', *Hastings Center Report* 7/2, 40–42.
40. Ramsey, P.: 1977, '"Euthanasia" and Dying Well Enough', *Lineacre Quarterly* 44 (February), 37–45.
41. Ramsey, P.: 1978, *Ethics at the Edges of Life: Medical and Legal Intersections*, Yale University Press, New Haven.
42. Ramsey, P.: 1978, 'Incommensurability and Indeterminacy in Moral Choice', in R.A. McCormick and P. Ramsey (eds.), *Doing Evil to Achieve Good: Moral Choice in Conflict Situations*, Loyola University Press, Chicago, pp. 69–144.
43. Ramsey, P.: 1981, 'Two-Step Fantastic: The Continuing Case of Brother Fox', *Theological Studies* 42, 122–34.
44. Rawls, J.: 1955, 'Two Concepts of Rules', *Philosophical Review* 64, 3–32.
45. Reich, W.: 1976, 'An Inquiry Into "Quality of Life" Ethics' (unpublished paper delivered at a conference on spina bifida babies, Skytop, PA, May 4–7).
46. Smith, D.H.: 1993, 'On Paul Ramsey: A Covenant-Centered Ethic for Medicine', in A. Verhey and S.E. Lammers (eds.), *Theological Voices in Medical Ethics*, William B. Eerdmans, Grand Rapids, MI, pp. 7–29.

CHAPTER FOUR

STANLEY HAUERWAS:
CHARACTER, VISION, AND NARRATIVE IN MORAL LIFE

A word of explanation is necessary at this point in our study. For, the moral theory to be elucidated in this chapter represents something of a sea-change relative to those theories considered heretofore. We have already noted that Hauerwas differs from McCormick and Ramsey in his insistence upon the priority of considering moral agents' fundamental constitution, or character, as opposed to focusing upon the content of their specific decisions and action-guiding norms. Indeed, Hauerwas refers to *integrity*, rather than 'rational deliberation' or obedience to moral norms, as the keystone of moral life. He goes so far as to suggest that moral dilemmas or disagreements are what happens "when all else has been lost" – i.e., when the moral 'vision' of involved parties is so skewed by self-deception or lack of a communal 'narrative' that they lack the skill truthfully to see the situation for what it is and respond in a manner integral to their formed convictions and life plans. In a sense, then, Hauerwas's enterprise will appear to some to involve a consideration of just about every factor in agential choosing and doing *other than* the sorts of abstract 'values' or 'rules' we have considered thus far.

This means, moreover, that if we are to try to describe Hauerwas's ethical method at all, then we will have to broaden somewhat the notion of 'method' we have been using. For, we have been examining McCormick's and Ramsey's theories of moral *decision making*, and we have been able to do so through the philosophical models of teleology and deontology. But Hauerwas not only rejects both of these models as neither necessary nor sufficient foundations for Christian ethical theory; he also believes that both models focus our attention on the wrong starting points for ethical reflection. Instead, he insists again and again that our primary concern should be to articulate "how Christian convictions form *lives*." Or, put another way,

The task of Christian ethics is to help us see how our convictions *are* in themselves a morality. We do not first believe certain things about God, Jesus, and the church, and subsequently derive ethical implications from those beliefs. Rather our convictions embody our morality; our beliefs are our actions ... Our moral life is not comprised of beliefs plus decisions; our moral life is the process in which our convictions form our character to be truthful ([13], p. 16).

In short, Hauerwas does not reject the importance of reflection upon moral choice; but he insists that we must *first* attend to the personal and communal convictions and 'stories' which form our dispositions to choose in certain ways and which enable us to see when and where situations of moral choice exist in the first place.

Now, the above quotation attests to yet another difference between Hauerwas's ethical approach and those considered previously – namely, the specifically religious, perhaps even sectarian, nature of Hauerwas's arguments and explanations. McCormick and Ramsey are, of course, engaged in theological ethics; we have seen many of the ways in which their theological convictions have formed their moral theories. But they have also sought to explicate genuinely universalistic moral theories, theories whose persuasive appeal is not limited to the eyes of faith or to any particular historical Christian community. Recall, for example, McCormick's claim that the *ordo bonorum* can be apprehended prediscursively by all, or Ramsey's assumptions of convergence between the covenantal obligations derived from *agape* and those deduced from the 'natural' covenants we all experience. In contrast to these approaches, Hauerwas has sought more or less consistently to illustrate the substantive *distinctiveness* of Christian ethics. He disclaims any attempt to be "defensive" or "exclusionary," but he insists that "methodologically, ethics and theology can only be carried out relative to a particular community's convictions" ([12], p. 4).

Indeed, he admits some uneasiness at having his work termed "ethics" if that designation is considered apart from "theology"; for he considers himself a theologian, and his work as "theology proper." Moreover, because he is unwilling to separate moral perception from the communal narratives through which perception is formed, he is even willing to claim that his position manifests "a certain kind of relativism" (as opposed to universalistic absolutism). It should be clear, then, that the form of ethical reflection described in this chapter will draw us far away from the sorts of methodological disputes we have encountered thus far.

Now, before proceeding to an introductory exposition of Hauerwas's position, it should also be noted that the task of drawing together even his major themes is no easy one. This is due in part to his penchant for the essay as a primary mode of presentation. The great majority of his published volumes (and all those dealing with issues in medical ethics) are collections of essays, many of them first published as journal articles, which cover a wide range of methodological arguments, topical and polemical discussions, responses to critics, etc. There is some redundancy among these essays, but not much. The sheer number of new themes and ideas he has developed in essay form is, in a word, staggering. As a result, the overview of Hauerwas's agenda presented here will be necessarily sketchy. Readers already familiar with his extensive corpus may find significant themes omitted or given short shrift. But my primary purposes are simply to introduce the dominant themes in Hauerwas's work and their relations one to another, and to clarify his approach to moral reflection in order to make intelligible his views on the three prismatic medico-moral issues which we are examining for comparative purposes.

Let us turn, then, to a consideration of Hauerwas's understanding of moral life, to be followed by sections devoted to his views on treatment-refusal by competent patients, treatment decisions for defective newborns, and the use of children in medical experimentation.

1. THE MORAL SELF IN STORIED COMMUNITY

This chapter's title suggests the primacy of three interrelated themes in Hauerwas's work: the *character* of moral agents; the moral *vision* necessary for forming and determining agential character; and the *stories* or *narratives* conveyed by particular communities or traditions, in and through which our visions of our world, who we are and want to become, etc., can be made intelligible.

Perhaps the best point of entry into all of this is Hauerwas's understanding of the agent-self and the formation of character. To speak of the idea of character, he writes, "is to recognize that our actions are also acts of self-determination; in them we not only reaffirm what we have been but also determine what we will be in the future." We not only shape particular situations through our actions; we also "form ourselves to meet future situations in a particular way" ([4], p. 49). Indeed, to be a human *person* is to be "an autonomous center of activity and the source of one's own determinations" ([5], p. 18). This idea of self-agency is central to the notion of character, and to stress the significance of character is to be "normatively committed to the idea that it is better for men to shape rather than to be shaped by their circumstances" ([5], p. 17). Put even more sharply, one is "at the mercy of external forces only if he allows himself to be" ([4], p. 55).

This is certainly a strong sense of agency! On the other hand, though, Hauerwas also insists that it does not deny those aspects of a person's life we think of as his/her 'destiny.' For, our possibilities are not unlimited; our range of choices is limited by particularities of social and cultural setting, our biographical and psychological situations, etc. Even so, it is yet the case that persons can gain character – which Hauerwas defines as "the orientation we give to our lives by ordering our desires, affections, and actions according to certain reasons rather than others" ([5], p. 203) – by responding with consistency and integrity to events beyond their own control. And, as Aristotle pointed out so long ago, we do hold persons accountable for what sort of persons they become – their character is a fit subject for praise or blame. So, while it may be that the agency of some persons is virtually crippled by the life-circumstances in which they find themselves, Hauerwas nevertheless insists that his notion of the self rests "metaphysically" on the "irreducible difference between what happens to a man and what he does" ([4], p. 56).

This is not to say, however, that we *create* our beliefs and convictions *de novo* on the way to forming and explaining our character and our behavior.

On the contrary, we are born into particular communities and inherit certain communal ways of viewing the world and describing what is going on in it. Moreover, Hauerwas insists upon the "essential sociality" of human 'nature'; action and agency are socially dependent by their very nature.[1] So, while denying that persons are necessarily *determined* by their societies "in the strong sense of the term," he is also denying that we can or should "become whatever we wish" ([4], p. 61). We cannot simply be formed passively by our community, but we are dependent upon it for the basic convictions and metaphors which provide our 'options' in seeing who we really are and want to become.

Now, there is, to be sure, no little tension between the claim that our moral development (in both cognitive and normative dimensions) is socially *dependent*, on the one hand, and the claim that our moral formation is *not* socially *determined*, on the other. Gene Outka has pointed out that Hauerwas is unclear about where the lines between human agency and human sociality might be drawn [29]. Hauerwas insists that the agent-self is never simply the product of social forces, and that "an unbridgeable gulf" exists between what I do and what happens to me. Yet, he also expresses great sympathy with G. H. Mead's "social conception of the self" [see note 1, above] and avers that his own emphasis on character "does not deny the basic dependence of the agent's determination upon society" ([5], p. 103, n. 25). In Outka's view, then, Hauerwas has failed to deal with the question of whether his "nearly unqualified appropriation" of Meadian social psychology may not in fact jeopardize his distinctive claims about character and self-agency ([29], p. 112).

Interestingly, Hauerwas agrees with Outka that the agency/sociality tension is present in his work, and he admits to a lingering uncertainty about how to resolve that tension. But he also believes that both sides of the tension need to be affirmed in *any* adequate account of moral life. His own view is that we should approach the issue by asking about the *kind* of agency made possible "through the way particular narratives teach us to see and be." Put in different terms, this means that "we can never remove our dependency, but we can integrate our dependency into a more determinative character" ([12], p. 257, n. 17). Obviously, such a restatement of the matter neither strengthens nor weakens the descriptive tension we have been considering. What it does, though, is to highlight what Hauerwas takes to be the characteristic mode of moral discernment by agents, through which agents can be said to be socially "dependent": namely, *vision*.

Morality, Hauerwas tells us, is not first and foremost a matter of *doing*, but rather of *seeing*. "The basis and aim of the moral life is to see the truth, for only as we see correctly can we act in accordance with reality" ([4], p. 102). Likewise, the primary task of the 'ethicist' is to help us discover the "essential metaphors" through which we can best see and understand our condition ([4], p. 30). In this interpretation of moral discernment Hauerwas follows closely upon the work of the British philosopher-novelist Iris Murdoch. Miss Murdoch has long argued that contemporary analytic (and existential) philosophy is built upon a much-too-grand understanding of human rationality and freedom; that human beings actually are unable to face the realities of our situation, and thus we tend to be defined by our illusion-making; and that philosophy manifests this symptom by attempting to break through the 'phenomenal' world to establish some necessary and perfect form and order.[2] So, philosophy has focused solely upon moral behavior as a matter of *choice*, and rational reasons for choice, when it is actually a matter of *vision*: "Our morality is more than adherence to universalizable rules; it also encompasses our experiences, fables, beliefs, images, concepts, and inner monologues" ([4], p. 35).

Building on these suggestions, Hauerwas constructs a notion of Christian ethics which involves not just decision-making but "learning 'to see' the world under the mode of the divine." We cannot separate our 'attending' the world as Christians from the distinctive language and metaphors that form Christian faith and tradition. The truth-claim of Christianity is that our particular language "actually envisages the world as it is." Thus, the morally important matter for the Christian is "transforming the self to fit the language," or "to become as we see" ([4], p. 46). Character is formed as we learn to see, for truthful vision is a *skill* which must be developed; we are, after all, by nature creators and lovers of illusion and self-deception. Moreover, Hauerwas avers, we are not really *free* until we learn to overcome the self-deception and self-absorption clouding our vision of reality. In this respect, the capacity to *love* can be seen as the condition necessary to real freedom, and the virtue of *humility* can be seen as freedom's most necessary habit or disposition ([4], p. 50).

Clearly, too, the skill of free and truthful vision is something attained not just personally but socially. One of Hauerwas's central theses in *A Community of Character*, for instance, is that human 'freedom' comes only "by participation in a truthful polity capable of forming virtuous people" ([12], pp. 2–3). Now, this manifests a decided change in emphasis from the strong claims of self-agency alluded to earlier. For here the self's agential freedom is described as a *result* of having one's visionary skills formed and directed through communal images and convictions rather than as the *condition* for self-determination of one's character. Indeed, Hauerwas's later definition of 'free' human agency makes this shift most clear:

Our 'freedom' . . . is dependent on our being initiated into a truthful narrative, as in fact it is the resource from which we derive the power to 'have character' at all . . .
   . . . [C]laims of agency are not meant to guarantee absolute freedom or independence. Freedom, or agency, is not a name for some real or ideal state in which we have absolute control of our lives. Rather 'agency' is but the word we use to remind us that we are beings who have the capacity to claim our lives by learning to grow in a truthful narrative ([13], p. 43).

Now, these statements represent a refinement of Hauerwas's earlier anthropological claim that persons are social by their very 'nature.' For here that very sociality is defined as the basis for the possibility of our expanded vision (and resultant descriptive ability). We are also told that our existence is social because it is *narrative* by nature. In other words, we apprehend the meaning of existence and of the world around us through stories – stories we learn in community and then assimilate ourselves into. Stories do not just illustrate or symbolize meaning for us; rather, they embody it in their very form ([10], p. 77). This is a crucial claim for Hauerwas's enterprise because, put in traditional terms, it means that human 'nature' is not 'rationality' itself but instead "the necessity of having a narrative to give our life coherence" ([10], p. 27). Given this assumption, his arguments against contemporary ethical theory become clearer. For, he contends that our familiar, analytic theories of moral obligation – e.g., teleological and deontological theories, all of which he lumps together as "the standard account" – have sought to make ethics an objective rational science through which we can apprehend universal truth and objective norms (available from any and every person's *rational* point of view). In the search for 'objectivity' in moral life, however, the presumption is that moral agents must be freed from (or transcend) their own 'subjective' stories – i.e., their own substantive historical, spatio-temporal frameworks for interpreting and describing the world. What the standard account fails to see, in Hauerwas's view, is that all our interpretive notions, including the notion of objective rationality itself, are narrative-dependent ([10], p. 21). If we try to abstract our search for the right, the good, the ideal, etc. from the stories (and narrative-dependent language) through which we apprehend and interpret reality in the first place, we are in fact attempting to lift ourselves out of our own history (which we cannot do) and we are creating for ourselves an a-historical and character-less isolation of the self. Moreover, the standard account's emphasis on rational judgement in moral *quandaries* is misplaced, since "it is character, inasmuch as it is displayed by a narrative, that provides the context necessary to pose the terms of a decision, or to determine whether a decision should be made at all" ([10], p. 20).

One immediate critical response to all of this might be that it smacks of moral relativism; and relativistic or subjectivistic moral judgement is precisely what the "standard account" has sought to avoid. Hauerwas admits that his account of moral life manifests "a certain kind of relativism" but not "a viscious relativism" ([12], p. 101). He is willing to say, for example, that certain things should be required of all people, regardless of their personal commitments, in "good societies" ([7], p. 648). And he allows that the principle of universalizability (as a criterion for moral principles) embodies the fundamental moral commitment "to regard all men as constituting a basic moral community"; it is thus a condition "without which moral argument and judgement are not possible" ([4], p. 85). But he also insists that the principle of universalizability as *the* hallmark of moral rationality simply cannot do what some philosophers and theologians wish it to do ([7], p. 650). For, the fact remains that, as Hauerwas puts it, "ethics always requires an adjective or qualifier" – e.g., Jewish, Hindu, Christian, existentialist, utilitarian, etc. (see [13], chapts. 1 and 2). This means simply that any response to basic moral questions – the nature of the right or good, of human freedom, etc. – necessarily draws upon the convictions of particular moral communities, for whom these questions may have different meanings ([13], p. 1). Indeed, 'morality' per se amounts to "the ongoing experience or conversation of a people that enables them to have a history sufficient for community identity" ([12], p. 102). Our very way of communicating about what is 'moral,' not to mention what is morally normative, emerges from the experiential narratives of our communities. (This means, too, that our most important moral convictions "are like the air we breathe: we never notice them because our life depends on them" – [13], p. 4.)

So, in Hauerwas's estimation, what we really need is not some decisive a priori argument against relativism, anyway; what we need is rather "an interpretation of and the corresponding skills to live in a world where others exist who do not share my moral history" ([12], p. 105). In other words, we need to be initiated into a communal narrative which allows us to see truthfully, even while admitting that our story may not be the only true story. Hauerwas appears to admit that, in this sense, Christian narratives may have no unique claim on moral truthfulness. Indeed, the truthfulness of any story lies in its capacity to form persons of clear and honest vision, not in its possession of absolute, universal and 'objective' truth-statements:

For morally there is no neutral story that insures the truthfulness of our particular stories. Moreover, any ethical theory that is sufficiently abstract and universal to claim neutrality would not be able to form character. For it would have deprived itself of the notions and convictions which are the necessary conditions for character . . . If truthfulness . . . is to be found, it will have to occur in and through the stories that tie the contingencies of our life together ([10], p. 24).

Because Hauerwas engages so frequently in describing and defending the moral truthfulness of distinctively *Christian* stories, it is easy for us to lose sight of the functional (and, in that respect, relativistic) form of his definition of a truthful story per se. But we should give careful attention to that definition. For, if a moral tradition (e.g., the Christian moral life) is indeed "determined more by the language we have learned to speak than by the decisions we make" ([6], p. 409), then it certainly makes a world of difference *which* moral language we accept as truthful. And if, as we saw above in Hauerwas's view of self-agency, we are in some sense *responsible* for shaping our own character (and vision) even as we are being shaped by our traditions and environments, then it would seem to follow that we are in some sense responsible for judging or choosing among the truthfulness-claims of various traditions or communities. To put it bluntly, the agency/sociality dialectic can be reduced no further than this: we are responsible for our own recognition and acceptance of the truthfulness of communal stories, even though our very ability to experience 'truthfulness' is mediated by the language of the communities which have shaped us.

Is there any point of entry into this apparent hermeneutical circle? Are there any *criteria* by which we might judge among alternative stories? Hauerwas suggests that there are. Specifically, he writes, any story we adopt, or allow to adopt us, should display:
(1) power to release us from destructive alternatives;
(2) ways of seeing through current distortions;
(3) room to keep us from having to resort to violence; [and]
(4) a sense for the tragic: how meaning transcends power ([10], p. 35).

A fifth criterion, cited separately as a condition of any "truthful tradition," is that tradition's recognition that it is not final, that it "needs to grow and change if it is to adequately shape our futures in a faithful manner" ([13], p. 45).

These criteria are not, as Hauerwas points out, features to be displayed in a story's content as such; rather, they refer to the expected *effect* of stories in shaping human persons. And he admits that such criteria will probably not pass "an impartial inspection." Nevertheless, he defends the above as realistic "working criteria." So, perhaps a few reflective comments about them would be in order at this point.

The first, second, and fourth criteria are rather straightforward expressions of what we have already seen of Hauerwas's description of character-formation and the significance of vision. Character development stems from our capacity to see and describe accurately (and beyond the distortions of ideology, self-absorption, etc.) the realities which surround us. Further, such clear vision involves a genuine appreciation of tragedy[3] in our lives: we must learn to see and express the deeper meanings of those realities we are powerless to transform into that which seems valuable to us. (This is a part of Hauerwas's critique of consequentialist moral theories, since they focus so exclusively on the 'goods' to be produced by human powers and interventions. In a similar vein, he insists that we must come to see medicine as a truly tragic profession, which means that we must learn to focus on the care possible when technological cure is not. The story of technology – of "setting nature aright" – simply cannot speak truthfully or meaningfully to the medical realities of human finitude and suffering.)

The fifth criterion of a truthful tradition or narrative – that it must be open to growth and change – is a bit more cryptic. The importance of this condition as a hedge against narrow, self-aggrandizing ideologies, or against the temptation to see one's own tradition as totally a-historical, is clear enough. But if the truthfulness-test of any tradition's story is "the sort of person it shapes," then what sort of "growth" or "change" in the directedness of human character(s) is to be counted as revelatory of a truthful story? (This is, admittedly, our original hermeneutical circle, viewed from a different angle.)

Perhaps the import of this question would be clearer if we ask more specifically about the significance of a tradition's "growth" and "change" in relation to the final remaining criterion of its truthfulness: that it display "room to keep us from having to resort to violence." First of all, what exactly does this latter condition require? What is its substantive stringency? Does it mean simply that a truthful narrative forms persons who will habitually seek, or try to create, non-violent solutions for human conflicts? Or does it also mean that truthful stories must form persons who will eschew, and avoid any participation in, acts or policies of violence, period? In other words, just how strict and categorical a commitment to nonviolence counts as evidence of the truthfulness of the communal narrative which gave rise to it?

Hauerwas never offers a clear answer to this – or at least no more specific, meta-traditional or meta-narrative criterion. He does, however, devote considerable attention to the non-violence engendered by the narratives of his own (truthful) tradition, Christianity (see, e.g., [13], [14], [17], [20], [22]). Indeed, Hauerwas is adamant that Christianity is inherently and necessarily pacifist. The Church's debate between pacifism and just war thinking, he writes, has been based upon differing understandings of history and its relation to God's kingdom; while war is a necessary and morally purposive part of *societies'* histories, those histories simply "are not God's history" ([14], p. 195). In other words, as Hauerwas sees it, any Christian theology which admits the option of war as an imaginable way of remedying the injustices of history is, to that extent at least, unfaithful to Christianity's storied history and eschatology.[4]

Now, given Hauerwas's particular interpretation of the Christian story, it certainly meets his non-violence criterion as a truthful narrative. But how do we *know* that the "living tradition" of Christianity must be pacifist in order to be faithful to its own (ongoing) story,[5] especially when we also know that the tradition has been kept "alive" for so many centuries by a community which has been predominantly non-pacifist? If Hauerwas's conception of the human self were more like Kant's, wherein all persons can partake rationally in a "noumenal" realm of objective truth transcending their own historical viewpoints, then he might argue that the pacifist position is one such objective truth which has been (for whatever reasons) insufficiently recognized for these many centuries. But, as we have seen, Hauerwas's understanding of the self is radically different from that. It focuses instead on "truth" as it is perceived and lived out in history and as we are *taught* to recognize it in and through historical communities. Given that vantage point, then just how do we *learn* to *see* that the greater part of Christendom has been self-deceived about Christianity's inherent pacifism (at least since the fifth century C.E.)?

Of course, one avenue of response open to Hauerwas at this point would be to refer us to his "growth and change" criterion for truthful stories. He might argue, for instance, that the Church's theological imagination has been focused on just-war thinking in the past not simply because of spiritual myopia or self-absorption with short-term human ends; rather, the just-war tradition could be seen as part of a gradual evolution or "growth" in the Church's ability to see clearly the reality of God's history. Such a response would keep us from having to say that the tradition in which we have learned to 'see' has been substantially untruthful in its own theological vision. But it would also raise another question of clarification for Hauerwas's list of criteria: If a truthful tradition must recognize that it is "not final" but needs to grow and change, then is it not possible that a truthful tradition could grow and change not only *toward* a position of non-violence but also *away from it*? Or, on the other hand, does Hauerwas's non-violence criterion for truthful stories somehow stand outside his growth-and-change criterion as a universal (and more-or-less absolute) standard? And, if so, how do we recognize it as such a universal standard?

From what has been said thus far, it should be clear that either answer creates potential complications for Hauerwas's conception of us as persons whose vision is formed by our traditions but who are nevertheless capable of recognizing the relative truthfulness or deceptiveness of those traditions.

Now, Hauerwas has presented much of the substance of his argument about the moral significance of character, vision, and truthful narrative in the form of extended examples, both positive and negative.[6] And the remaining sections of this chapter will follow that pattern by examining how he has approached the concrete issues of medical treatment-refusal, treatment choices for handicapped infants, and children's participation in medical experiments. Before turning to those illustrative examples, however, we should note two other, central facets of Hauerwas's work: his strong critique of modern 'liberal' ideologies, and his emphasis on the Church's critical role as a community of "resident aliens" within liberal society.

The ethos of liberalism is premised upon the primacy of individual freedom – freedom to pursue one's own values or interests (while not violating the freedom of others to pursue theirs). Implicit in this is an assumption that individual value-commitments, and the stories which form them, are quite diverse in our society. As Hauerwas interprets it,

Liberalism is successful exactly because it supplies us with a myth that seems to make sense of our social origins. For there is some truth to the fact that we originally existed as a people without any shared history, but came with many different kinds of histories. In the absence of any shared history we seemed to lack anything in common that could serve as a basis for societal cooperation. Fortunately, liberalism provided a philosophical account of society designed to deal with exactly that problem: A people do not need a shared history; all they need is a system of rules which will constitute procedures for resolving disputes as they pursue their various interests. Thus liberalism is a political philosophy committed to the proposition that a social order and a corresponding mode of government can be formed on self-interest and consent ([12], p. 78).

The irony in all this, Hauerwas tells us, is that the founders of American liberal polity also assumed a virtuous people. In other words, they believed that some more-or-less common understanding of what we should *do* with our freedom would (and must) shape our public character – not just the fact that we are free to pursue competing interests. But what has developed has been the reverse of this: our so-called "private morality" has followed the form of our public polity, and the original *premise* of personal freedom has become the singular *end* of liberal theory. As a result, liberalism becomes "a self-fulfilling prophecy; a social order that is designed to work on the presumption that people are self-interested tends to produce that kind of people" ([12], p. 79).

Moreover, this result becomes a counsel of despair for Americans who want to be 'good people' but have "lost any idea of what that could possibly mean." Indeed, in terms of any narrative understanding of 'goodness' in ourselves and the world, liberalism is formally 'neutral.' But that, in Hauerwas's view, is its most coercive aspect. For, in describing a world in which we are "free to make up our own story," liberalism teaches us that we have no story. And that is a story in itself – one whose deep determination of our lives we fail to notice ([12], p. 84). The perspective we develop is one of individualism and isolation, which we have learned to call "autonomy" or "freedom" to mask the fact that it is really *loneliness* ([12], p. 81). As examples of the isolation of selves inherent in liberal 'rights' language, Hauerwas cites the notions of a "right to have children" and the "rights of children" against their parents. What understanding of "family" can possibly emerge from such language, except perhaps that of a "contractual society"? (This line of criticism will be developed further in later sections of this chapter.)

Given this dark view of liberalism as engendering self-interest, isolation, and, ultimately, distrust among individuals, and given the fact that "our society offers no ready alternatives to liberalism," then where can we look for the source of anything like "public virtue"? Hauerwas's response is that the Church, through its own example, must challenge the presumptions of liberalism. While liberalism teaches us that we can have no authority except that which we ourselves have freely instituted, the church is a community cognizant of the need for authority in all societies, political and religious. Further, the Church's constitution "takes the form of the story of a savior who taught us to deal with power by recognizing how God limits all earthly claims to power"; thus, the Church can eschew any earthly claims to power and provide the world with an example of how to live non-violently.

Because Christians know that the story of God is the truthful narrative of our own existence, we can and must be a community founded on trust rather than on distrust and simple self-interest. The church's first social task, then, is to "be herself" (and, in so doing, to avoid conflating the Christian story with any historical polity). For, only by witnessing to our own story and its authority can the church "exhibit in our common life the kind of community possible when trust, and not fear, rules our lives" ([12], p. 85).

Many of Hauerwas's more recent essays and books have dealt with the question of what it *means* for the Church to "be herself" within society. And many respondents have taken issue with what they interpret as his call for the Church's separation from the world. Hauerwas claims, for instance, that the Church must be a "colony," which he defines as ". . . a beachhead, an outpost, an island of one culture in the middle of another, a place where the values of home are reiterated and passed on to the young, a place where the distinctive language and life-style of the resident aliens are lovingly nurtured and reinforced" ([24], p. 12). And he insists that the "political task" of Christians is *not* to "transform the world" but simply to "be the Church" ([24], p. 30). Such language has led some to accuse Hauerwas of "sectarianism," "tribalism," "fideism," or even "elitism." James Gustafson argues, for example, that Hauerwas's project has "wedded a way of doing theology – narratives – to an ecclesiology – classical sectarian – and to an ethic which is also classically sectarian" ([2], p. 88). And Martin Marty, citing H.R. Niebuhr's famous typology in *Christ and Culture*, observes that Hauerwas's ecclesiological paradigm is certainly "Christ against culture" [27].

Not surprisingly, Hauerwas vigorously denies such charges as misinterpretations of his enterprise. For, his aim is not to isolate the Christian community but to bring the Church back to its own story, which requires reminders about whose it is, how it came into being, and in whom alone its truth resides. And the major barrier to that return is the Church's modern "Constantinianism" – i.e., its identification with and accommodation to political agendas (on the left and the right) for social change/improvement, agendas which do not need or depend upon Jesus's story for their credibility. Moreover, agendas of social-political activism necessarily require expressions of worldly power, and thus are inherently coercive and violent; whereas the Church's truth is a non-violent truth, neither needing nor seeking worldly power. Hauerwas insists that he is not counseling Christians' disengagement from political, economic and social activities in society; he is counseling instead a radical re-prioritization of those activities in light of the Church's story. "The issue," he writes, "is how the Church can provide the interpretive categories to help Christians better understand the positive and negative aspects of their societies and guide their subsequent selective participation" ([17], p. 11).

Of course, if the Church is to provide "interpretive categories" for the faithful, then the next obvious question is, *Who* is doing the (initial) interpreting – who is speaking as/for the Church and its story? While Hauerwas's answer to this is not entirely clear, he does make it quite clear that interpretation of Christian narratives cannot be a 'liberal' or 'democratic' affair. The Christian community's primary narrative source – the Scripture – should, in Hauerwas's estimation, be "taken away from Christians in North America" ([20], p. 17). Reading Scripture correctly is not an 'objective' science or discipline; and, further, "the Church creates the meaning of Scripture" ([20], p. 36). Thus, the "right" reading of Scripture depends on having "spiritual masters" who can help the whole Church "stand under the authority of God's Word" ([20], p. 16). Apparently, then, individual Christians are to be formed in the Christian narratives through the hermeneutical readings (called "allegory" by Hauerwas) of those called to and trained in the Church's ministry of proclamation. (Hauerwas's notion of proper clerical authority has other dimensions, too. For instance, in *Resident Aliens* he and William Willimon raise the question of whether United Methodist pastors should deny admission to the Lord's Table to those who make a living building weapons [p. 160].)

Hauerwas admits that this understanding of ecclesial interpretive authority appears strange to many in North American churches, particularly those in liberal Protestant denominations. But he insists that if we are to understand Scripture, it is necessary that we "place ourselves under authority, a placement that at least begins by our willingness to accept the Church's preaching" ([20], p. 38). For many critics, of course, this view is problematic not just because it is clerically "elitist" but because it severely narrows the range of potential hermeneutical correctives in the quest for a narrative's truths by de-emphasizing the need to listen to "others" in the Church who are themselves struggling to live the Christian story. John Howard Yoder finds it "imperative to doubt" the wisdom of leaving interpretive authority to clergy alone, and James McClendon insists upon "a never-ending congregational conversation" for keeping the Church faithful. Reflecting on the differences between Hauerwas, Yoder and McClendon on this point, Gloria Albrecht argues that none of them really attends to the other fundamental, practical problem of interpretive "authority," namely, "the power relations that actually exist within church communities and the effective silencing of voices which might challenge the views they assume." Essentially, she writes,

the authority-of-clergy vs. authority-of-community debate ... conceals the reality that authority in either case lies within the hands of (predominantly white) male clerical or (predominantly white) male communal leadership. The obvious problematic consequence for women and for men of color is that an authentic understanding of scripture requires submission to the authority and discipline of a (white) male dominated institutional church, its self-defined traditions, its seminaries, and its professional disciplines. Nonetheless, Hauerwas, Yoder and McClendon argue that only by this authority and under this discipline, Christians learn to 'see' their world. Without this authority, we do not 'see' as Christians ([1], Chapter 2).

Albrecht's concerns about power relations within the Church, and their consequences for interpretive authority, would apply not only to present, ongoing interpretive activity in the Church but also to its received "traditions" of interpretation. For, the power relations to which she alludes are, frankly, as old as the Church itself. Hauerwas does not (to my knowledge) address the problem of power-preserving 'slant' in interpretation (or interpretive tradition), despite his assertion that all interpretation is "an exercise in politics." And I doubt that he would entertain it as a 'problem' at all. For, he asserts simply (and with great confidence) that Scriptural texts have no "real meaning" in and of themselves; that the Church "creates" the meaning of Scripture "in the form of some in the Church reminding others in the Church how to live as Christians"; and that, in the interpretive process, "the Church, through the guidance of the Holy Spirit, tests contemporary readings of Scripture against the tradition, knowing that such readings help us to see the limits of the present" ([20], pp. 28, 36, 37). In Hauerwas's repeated (indeed, constant) claims about how "the Church" interprets and proclaims the truths of Scripture, he appears to be referring to the interpretive/proclamatory work of those "spiritual masters" within the Church. Whatever 'slant' those persons might bring to the hermeneutical process does not seem to be a relevant concern to him, given the sort of "guidance" he believes them to have.

In any case, Hauerwas insists that the aim of "the Church's preaching" is to keep the Christian community "capable of living faithful by remembering well," which requires helping Christians to "extend our habits in ways not foreseen" ([20], p. 36). The Church is, then, a "school for virtue" within itself. But it can and must be also a school for virtue within society – especially since liberal culture can offer no truthful story to remember or to live faithfully within. The Church can accomplish that task by manifesting itself as a community that is

... the source for imaginative alternatives for social policies that not only require us to trust one another, but chart forms of life for the development of virtue and character as public concerns. The problem in liberal societies is that there seems to be no way to encourage the development of public virtue without accepting a totalitarian strategy from the left or an elitist strategy from the right. By standing as an alternative to each, the church may well help free our social imagination from those destructive choices. For finally social and political theory depends on people having the experience of trust rather than the idea of trust ([12], p. 86).

While this passage neatly summarizes many of Hauerwas's claims about the Church's role vis-à-vis modern liberal society, it also serves as a fitting introduction for the remainder of this chapter. For we will see, in the following sections, other specific illustrations of how, in Hauerwas's view, the Christian story can "help free our social imagination from . . . destructive choices." Let us turn our consideration, then, to some of his reflections concerning medical ethics issues.

110   CHAPTER FOUR

2. MORAL AGENCY, COMMUNITY, AND MEDICAL TREATMENT CHOICES FOR ONESELF

... [W]e must be careful not to get so taken up with securing a good death that we forget that our aim is to live. Death is not a romantic adventure; it is what we do not know and it is seldom pretty. The issue is not whether we have a 'right to die,' but whether we and our community are morally healthy and can face death in a spirit of human solidarity ([4], p. 181).

    This quotation introduces several of the major themes in Hauerwas's reflections on treatment refusals by competent patients which will be considered in this section: our attitudes toward suffering and death; the meaning of human 'freedom' and its relation to autonomous self-determination; and the reciprocal responsibilities between dying patients and the communities surrounding them. Hauerwas has not addressed the specific issue of treatment-refusal nearly so often as he has dealt with the related issue of suicide; and he rarely ventures into making specification as to which particular situations of treatment-refusal would constitute a choice for suicide. But his articles on suicide often include comments about refusals of life-prolonging treatment, and, as we will see, the lines of his argument do not so much depend upon the establishment of clear or 'objective' definitional boundaries, anyway.

    Perhaps we should begin with a few of his observations about the theological and human meaning of death. First of all, life, for Christians, is "not sacred in the strict sense." It is not to be considered an end in itself, but as a medium for service in God's kingdom. So, Christians "are not fundamentally concerned about living. Rather, their concern is to die for the right thing." Any attempt to construct a simple ideology of the 'sanctity of life' would misleadingly imply that Christians are committed to the proposition that "there is nothing in life worth dying for" ([16], p. 92).

    Nothing in Christianity, then, as Hauerwas sees it, suggests that medical preservation of life should be considered an indefeasible obligation or end in itself, whether that life be one's own or another's. "Rather, the Gospel demands the *care* of the weak, which is quite a different matter" ([4], p. 177). At the same time, however, Hauerwas asserts, with Ramsey, that Christians always maintain "the Jewish sense of the body's significance" ([16], p. 91). We cannot affirm any "higher aspects" of our being without also affirming that we have no further potential without our bodies ([4], p. 175). He also agrees with Ramsey that life must be considered a *gift*, but a gift for which we must care, as it provides our means for service. And indeed, one form of service incumbent upon us may well be "our willingness to stay alive amid the ambiguity and destructiveness of our existence," because others will then see this as a support and testimony that they, too, can go on living "in a hopeful and trustful manner." Thus, the moral commitments which sustain our lives together, and which we should exemplify, lead us to believe that we should express our willingness even to carry suffering rather than to seek death as a relief from it ([16], p. 36).

Undergirding these reflections is an understanding of death's meaning which Hauerwas calls "the realism of the New Testament" and which he associates with Pauline theology (although some of its particulars seem to have been drawn from strands of classical ontology as well). Basically, "death is not the worst thing that could happen to a Christian. But neither is it a good thing." In Hauerwas's reading, Paul also reminds us that "a Christian may desire death in a manner which denotes lack of trust in God's triumph over death" ([16], p. 96). Death is something to be feared and avoided, but this is so precisely because death's contribution to our lives is not only negative but also *positive*:

Without death our lives would have no height or depth, for nothing is precious in a world that literally has time for everything. For example, death makes precious the ones I love by forcing me to regard them as finite beings . . . Death creates the economy that makes it necessary to choose between life projects, between that which is valuable and that which is not. As such, death is a *precious gift* which we cannot live without ([4], p. 177f. – emphasis added).

Despite its giftedness, though, death cannot be embraced as friend because it eventually negates all those things it has taught us to love. So it is "at once friend and enemy, brother and stranger." Our theological affirmations thus must keep both polarities in view; otherwise they will distort our ability to see life as formed and destined by death ([4], p. 178). A proper fear of death should not be "perverted" into any ideology of the absoluteness of life, especially in the practice of medicine. At the other extreme, however, Christians must avoid any implication that the deaths of those close to us are somehow causes for celebration; that would be "false and pretentious faith." For,

It is God's prerogative to rejoice in the death of one of His own, but He can do that because He is God. By His grace we do not have to try to be like God; thus death for us is rightly an occasion of grief and sadness. To treat it otherwise is to rob death of its human significance. Of course the sadness of the Christian is bounded by hope, but such hope is only truthful when it takes seriously the reality of death as acute separation from the human community ([4], pp. 181–82).

With all this in mind, then, Hauerwas reminds us that Christian faith offers a hopeful and also *truthful* means for understanding our reality – including the reality of *tragedy* in our lives. What was for the Greeks the notion of 'fate' has been transformed in the Christian tradition to *gift* or *grace*. And our learning how to accept a gift (such as life or death) puts us on the road to becoming good persons insofar as it gives us a moral basis for understanding that we are under the power not of indifferent fate but of Providence ([10], p. 200).

It is because we have lost the moral importance of the sense of gift that we are lacking the skill to deal with tragedy. We must learn to see, though, that medicine is indeed a tragic profession, as it "reflects the very limits of our existence" ([10], p. 190). What medicine needs for its moral empowerment is a community – something like the Church, Hauerwas suggests – that can provide ways of seeing the truth about suffering, death, and tragedy and allow us to *care* where cure is not possible ([16], pp. 63–82). Otherwise, medicine will continue to succumb to the death-denying and death-avoiding illusions so common in our society and we will continue to expect physicians to be "priests of the new magic." Or, alternatively, medicine may be "grasped by another set of convictions that promises more than it can ever deliver, namely, the attempt to insure autonomy as an end in itself" ([10], p. 196).

This latter possibility – the acceptance of 'autonomy' as an end or goal – is a frequent target of Hauerwas's criticism. For, he sees it as the result of our self-deceptive absorption with liberal individualism. So, let us turn again to his reflections about moral agency, freedom, and 'autonomy.' As we have seen in the previous section, there is some tension between Hauerwas's notions of agency as forming the self through its choices and as being formed by the self's community and its stories. At the risk of possible redundancy, though, we need to look a bit more closely at the various faces of "free agency" in his corpus, in order better to understand his views about treatment choices made by patients for themselves.

In the 'early' Hauerwas (particularly *Character and the Christian Life* and *Vision and Virtue*), very strong connections are made between the practice of self-determination and being a 'person' at all:

[M]en are *in essence self-determining beings*, who act upon and through their environment to give their lives particular form . . . To be a man is to be an *autonomous center of activity* and the source of one's own determinations ([5], p. 18 – emphases added).

Moreover, to be *free* is, likewise, "to set a course through the multitude of possibilities that confront us and so impose order on the world and ourselves."[7]

Now, this is a definitional line which is certainly familiar in moral philosophy (and theology, for that matter). It is also the basis for Hauerwas's ascription of moral responsibility to all persons for what they choose and do in the process of becoming and expressing who they are. However, it is not a normative claim for pure self-legislation; the self's autonomy "is not a status to be assumed but a task to be undertaken." And freedom is not "the will jumping from one isolated instance to another." Indeed, the "correlate" of freedom is not the will at all; it is instead "the *truth* of our intention" ([4], p. 65).

In one of Hauerwas's earliest essays on the issues of suicide and euthanasia (with Richard Bondi) the authors examine those two issues in terms of attitudes toward *life* rather than toward special cases of death ([10], pp. 101–15). They suggest that *memory* is a prized virtue since our lives must be formed (and our decisions guided) by the stories which truthfully "capture our past, sustain our present, and give our future direction." Forgetfulness, then, is a sort of vice; forgetfulness about who we are as a people, "created by a God who sets our way" is indeed what we call "sin" ([10], p. 104f.) In light of this, the problem with suicide is not that it may not be 'free' or 'autonomous,' but that it "eradicates the presence of the other and results in the other's loss in our memory." Our very willingness to exist – to be present with and for each other – has a profound moral significance as part of the truth we should be free to know. For, one of the truths of the Christian story is that life is "the gift of time enough for love" ([10], pp. 106–7). Moreover, the form of our death can help affirm symbolically the network of trust we need, and need to offer, in life; and it should also provide for "healthful and morally sound grief" (and memory) for those we leave behind ([10], pp. 110–11).

Having said all this, Hauerwas and Bondi also point out that affirming the trustworthiness of God's care also means accepting the "fatedness" of our ending. And (in rather uncharacteristic language) they insist that "dying" persons have "a right to refuse medical care."[8] Citing the example of renal dialysis, they claim that there is no obligation to use it, "especially when we are old and few depend on us. We have the right to die as we have lived." Even so, this "right" extends only to refraining from acting (or not accepting medical treatment) and not to active interventions to bring about death. Holding to this distinction[9] in such cases illustrates to the one who suffers "the continuing trustworthiness of his or her existence" ([10], p. 115).

This instance of rights-language, with its ostensible connotations of individual self-determination, finds little support in the bulk of Hauerwas's later work.[10] Indeed, *A Community of Character* is in large part a critique of liberal rights-theory and its ideology of 'autonomy.' For, such an ideology isolates us in self-deceptive egoism, whereas the true "freedom" of persons "comes only by participation in a truthful polity capable of forming virtuous people" ([12], p. 2f.) The Christian, formed by narratives of the Christian community, seeks neither 'independence' nor 'autonomy.' He seeks instead to be "faithful to the way that manifests the conviction that we belong to another." This is why we describe our lives as 'gifts' rather than 'achievements' ([12], p. 130). Hauerwas allows that this will sound like a form of "heteronomy" to many post-Kantian philosophers; but he insists that what *they* mean by "autonomous freedom" can mean for the Christian only slavery to self and self-desire. Freedom itself is "literally a gift" for Christians, since it comes by "being accepted as disciples and thus learning to imitate a master." We learn *how* we are to do what we must do only by watching and following ([12], p. 131).

This understanding of agential freedom as an imitative task finds further development in *The Peaceable Kingdom*, where Hauerwas elaborates on the relation between freedom and the community's narratives:

My act is not something I cause, as though it were external to me, but it is mine because I am able to 'fit' it into my ongoing story. My power as an agent is therefore relative to the power of my descriptive ability. Yet that very ability is fundamentally a social skill, for we learn to describe through appropriating the narratives of the communities in which we find ourselves ([13], p. 42).

This means that our freedom is "literally in the hands of others," because it is from others that we learn the stories that give our lives purpose and direction. Moreover, it is the *needs* of others which help us to render irrelevant the greatest hindrance to our freedom, namely, self-absorption ([13], pp. 44–45). For these reasons, Hauerwas refers to freedom as "the presence of the other."

With these various reflections on human agency as background, then, let us turn to a consideration of Hauerwas's more developed reflections on suffering and choices for death, collected in *Suffering Presence*.

One of the themes receiving considerable attention in that volume is, of course, *suffering*. Hauerwas suggests that perhaps the "most decisive challenge" medicine raises for Christian convictions and morality "involves the attempt to make suffering pointless and thus subject to elimination." Certainly suffering tends to alienate us from others and from ourselves, but it is "exactly the ability to make the suffering mine that is crucial if I am to be an integral self" ([16], pp. 24–25) Indeed, while some have argued that medicine's primary purpose should be to relieve our suffering because that suffering robs us of our autonomy, Hauerwas contends that we can *gain* our autonomy only by our willingness to make our suffering our own "through its incorporation into our moral projects." This is because 'autonomy,' as Hauerwas defines it, is correlative to our having a narrative within which we can incorporate even suffering as part of our own true story ([16], p. 33f.). So, while we should not *welcome* suffering, and while it may indeed be a test of our character, we would be mistaken – at least within the Christian story – to make medical treatment decisions on the basis of calculations of how much suffering is preferable to death. "Rather our decisions must turn on what we think our lives are for, and not how much suffering they contain or how long we can avoid death" ([16], p. 35).

Moreover, Hauerwas suggests that part of our problem in considering care for dying patients has been that we have neglected to consider the kind of responsibilities those patients have themselves. The dying indeed have obligations to the living. Among these obligations is the responsibility "to die well." A patient "too willing to die" can make those around him feel that their own lack of care has led him to leave life "without wishing to retain anything." Instead, his manner of death should be morally commensurate with the kind of trust which has sustained him heretofore; others should see that they are sustaining him and that God is given due credit as the ultimate giver of life ([16], p. 96). Moreover, as Hauerwas points out in a critique of suicide, the obligations of sick and dying persons do not entail any sort of calculation of the 'burdensomeness' of their care:

> We fear being a burden for others, but even more to ourselves. Yet it is only by recognizing that in fact we are inescapably a burden that we face the reality and opportunity of living truthfully ([16], p. 107).

Thus our dying, like our living, should be formed by the community's story which has become our own, and it should express the truths of that story — particularly our trustful dependence upon God and one another.

But along with his claim that our willingness to live is "morally a service to one another," Hauerwas also reminds us once again that life is not inherently sacred and that we need not do everything possible to keep ourselves alive in all conditions. He expresses some sympathy with attempts to distinguish morally between 'preserving life' and 'only prolonging dying,' but he is not willing to concur with Ramsey that this distinction is a purely medical determination: ". . . such a distinction does not turn on technical judgements about when we have in fact started dying, though it may involve such a judgment . . . Rather the distinction is dependent on the inherited wisdom of a community that has some idea of what a 'good death' entails" ([16], p. 106; see also p. 33 and [4], p. 183f.).

Consistent with his intent to consider life-and-death medical choices within a framework of storied attitudes and commitments rather than from the perspective of physicians' and patients' obligations and rights, Hauerwas's reflections resist any simple reinterpretation within the ongoing debate about 'patient autonomy' vs. 'medical paternalism.' And this is deliberate on his part. For, he sees both (vitalistic) medical paternalism and the ideology of patients' rights as symptoms of the same basic problem: the lack of any shared story and ethos in our society that can offer us a common wisdom about the meanings of life, death, suffering, finitude, and authority. He does suggest that a community's general refusal to let an attempted suicide die constitutes an attempt, however feeble, to "remain a community of trust and care through the agency of medicine." For, by prohibiting suicide and caring for those who attempt it, we draw on "our profoundest assumptions that each individual's life has a purpose beyond simply being 'autonomous'" ([16], p. 107).

As to the specific issue of how medicine should respond to terminally ill patients' treatment choices, Hauerwas seems to come closest to an actual policy recommendation in one of the essays in his first published volume, *Vision and Virtue*. So, perhaps we should conclude this section with that statement:

> . . . I would make the plea that the patient himself be consulted about his dying — namely, that his dying be considered not just a matter of when the physiological machinery is run down, but under what conditions he wants to place himself as it runs down. I think that this can and should vary from one person to another. Consistent with the life plan they have embodied in their character, some may wish to fight to the end, using all the available means of medical technology.

But others may form their death in quite a different way consistent with their character, not fighting but calmly accepting death as an affirmation of their willingness to provide a place for new life among us ([4], p. 184).

3. SUFFERING, DEATH, AND CARING FOR OUR CHILDREN: HAUERWAS ON NEONATAL TREATMENT DECISIONS

Another frequent locus of Hauerwas's consideration is our attitude toward, and care of, the mentally or physically handicapped – particularly handicapped children. The title of this section reflects those themes he brings to bear most often on questions of treatment for handicapped neonates: the reality and necessity of suffering and death, and the notion of parental (and medical) 'care' of children. Although he does offer some specific suggestions for decision making about treatment, he is – as always – more fundamentally concerned with the moral formation of persons who must make those decisions and the communities in which they are made. He insists, for example, that our basic moral question in such matters must be "what kind of families and communities should we be so we could welcome retarded children into our midst regardless of the happy or unhappy consequence they may bring" ([10], p. 147).

Let us begin, then, with some of his views on our attitudes toward having and rearing children. One of our basic problems, he writes, is that we have learned to see the begetting of children as a fundamental 'freedom' or 'right.' And our strong assumption that we indeed "choose" our children has made us claim an "unwarranted responsibility" for their well-being. We blame ourselves if their genetic make-up is somehow less than ideal or if they don't seem happy. But just as we assume such responsibility in our choosing, we also place a tremendous demand on children – namely, "that they be perfect." What we should have learned to see in our having and raising children, however, is that we really "disclose them as gifts that are not of our own making" ([10], pp. 149–50). Indeed, the Christian understanding of procreation draws on the profound conviction that God is Lord of the world, and that we can affirm the goodness of it and our existence in it – despite the misery we see in it – because we can affirm that God is creator and redeemer of it. In light of this, children are "our promissory note, our sign to present and future generations, that we Christians trust the Lord who has called us together to be his people" ([10], p. 151). Moreover, the sacrifice of the Son of God at Calvary reveals that even the weakest among us "are valued in ways not dependent on our human purposes and strengths" ([4], p. 189).

Learning to recognize our children as gifts has a powerful didactic function; for, genuine gifts *create needs* – that is, "they teach us what wants we should have, as they remind us how limited we are without them." In particular, children create in us the proper need to want to regard and love another; and they draw our love and regard while at the same time "refusing to be as we wish them to be." So, while creating our duties of love and care for them, they also teach us true *freedom* by helping us accept the proper limitations of being human ([10], p. 153).

Retarded and otherwise handicapped children are certainly special gifts. They remind us more quickly than most children that our plans for our progeny may not be commensurate with the true purpose for our having them. But their giftedness also reminds us that, whatever their particular burdens, they do not exist simply to make us feel better about ourselves for the sacrifices we may have to make, either:

I am not suggesting that Christians should rejoice that their children are born retarded rather than normal. Rather I am suggesting that as Christians the story that informs and directs why we have children at all provides us with the skill to know how to welcome these particular children into our existence without telling ourselves self-deceiving stories about our heroism for doing so. For such heroic stories can also serve to subject the retarded child to forms of care that they should not be forced to undergo ([10], p. 154).

Hauerwas seems to want to distinguish carefully between our willingness to care for handicapped children for the purpose of feeling or appearing 'heroic,' on the one hand, and as an expression of our humane commitments, on the other. For example, in his critique of various definitions of 'personhood' (as indicators of when we owe treatment to a given child) he insists that such definitions teach us very little about ethical presumption. "For the question is not whether [handicapped babies] are human persons, but rather what kind of care we should give them in order for us to be humane" ([10], p. 174f.). While the language here appears purposeful and self-referential, his point is that "humane" care can flow only from our learning that the opportunity to give special care to those "particularly at the mercy of the human predicament" is "an essential aspect of our humanity."

Hauerwas's strong critique of the ethos of "procreative freedom" rests upon a further presumption, too – that such an ethos blinds us to the reality and meaning of children's suffering. For, if we assume the freedom and the *responsibility* of guaranteeing a happy and successful life for our children, we also become inordinately concerned to spare our children from suffering. Ironically, this means that we often "reduce the options at birth to a perfect child or a dead child." But such an assumption about parenthood is "extraordinarily Promethean" and also false. We "cannot and should not raise our children as if they could be protected against suffering and death."[11] Besides, there is something truly odd about the very notion that death (for a defective baby) is better than a life of suffering – odd because it may lead us to eliminate the *sufferer* in order to eliminate the suffering ([16], p. 23f.). Moreover, the simple commitment to 'relieve suffering' can be self-deceptive. We need to be clear about *whose* suffering we are most concerned to end – the infant-patient's physical and mental pain or *our* pain at having to be "next to a patient we cannot relieve" ([10], p. 167). Finally, we must also bear in mind the practical reality that the willingness of health professionals to allow, and be present with, pain and suffering has been the precondition of most medical advances: "By our willingness to stand in the presence of such pain we create the conditions that impel the imagination to explore yet unthought forms of care."[12]

In sum, the suffering of our children is not a 'good' thing to be sought for them; it is rather something to be realistically accepted, in Christian hopefulness, as a condition of our finitude. The death of our children is likewise an inescapable reality, and in some circumstances a reality no longer to be put off; but the fact of their suffering is not in itself a morally sufficient reason for choosing to eliminate the sufferer in order to get rid of his/her suffering.

Now, if we are indeed formed by these understandings of our existence and our world, then under what circumstances might parents 'humanely' choose to forgo further life-prolonging treatments for a defective newborn? Hauerwas offers no list of particulars. But he does offer, in addition to his general reflections on parenting and suffering, some interpretive guidelines for neonatal treatment decisions. And he does so in the context of reflecting upon two other conceptual matters: the meaning of 'child' (especially vis-à-vis other attempts to define 'person' for moral purposes) and the supposed distinction between 'killing' and 'letting die.'

As we have seen, Hauerwas is critical of all definitions of 'person' which stipulate qualities to be attained before an individual can merit the full moral protections we afford each other, because this misses the question of what our "humane" attitudes should be. At one point, though, he does reformulate the question of whether certain defects might disqualify children as human 'persons' to the question of "whether these defects can materially alter the obligation we feel to care for them as fellow-sufferers who also are our children." And here his emphasis is not so much on *our* [parents' and caregivers'] "humanity," but instead on the human *relations* these children already *do have* with us. Note his wording: "fellow-sufferers," and "our children." These relational terms are significant in that they call attention to our conviction that defective newborns should be treated equal to others, to whom they are related, when it comes to life-and-death decisions. And Hauerwas insists that there is no reason "[i]n principle . . . why the defective newborn has any less claim to care than any newborn," even if we can find good philosophical reasons for claiming that he/she is not yet a 'person' ([10], p. 176). Yet, language employed to connote relationship usually implies also some common capacity or potential for relating or responding. And this implication certainly enters into Hauerwas's suggestion of when a defective child might *not* really be a 'child': ". . . I see no reason why these [handicapped] children's defects materially disqualify them from being children *unless their defect is so severe there is little possibility that they will ever be able to respond to care*"[13] ([10], p. 177 – emphasis added. Note the similarity between this obligation-limiting criterion and McCormick's corresponding criterion of "relational potential" [see Chapter 2]).

This capacity, then – the ability (or potential) to be responsive to care – seems to be for Hauerwas one fairly clear signpost for us in determining our parental responsibilities to provide treatment. And we must emphasize "parental" responsibilities here, for Hauerwas repeatedly expresses the notion of parenting as the nexus of all responsibility – societal, medical, etc. – toward the child. In reflecting on surgery-refusal cases like the Johns Hopkins case,[14] for instance, he allows that perhaps we should not argue for a parental/medical obligation to perform the surgery when there is no broader societal support for the handicapped baby. But he questions why the parents should be relieved of the responsibility of taking the baby home to die, if death is their decision. For, doctors do not have and should not accept the responsibility of watching the child die in order to spare the parents suffering; if they do, the parents "have no sense of the full reality of the decision they have made" ([10], pp. 167–68). It is not the doctor's task to help the parents avoid guilt in such matters. Moreover, Hauerwas insists (in a consideration of treatment for spina bifida babies) that the superior technical knowledge doctors have is not enough to justify keeping the parents from being the primary decision makers for their children, either. Perhaps parents have difficulty with the medical data, and perhaps they have difficulty imagining the problems their child will face; but these considerations are not decisive enough "to rob them of the right of making the decision" ([9], p. 241). Indeed, such considerations rather mandate more careful or well-rounded ways for doctors to impart information to parents (such as introducing them to other parents with similarly afflicted children).

Now, while insisting that parents are the proper agents of decision making, and that they should be able to see their responsibility to provide all necessary medical care for their children (or at least those who are or can be a 'child'), Hauerwas also goes on to call our attention to one other possible source of self-deception in these matters – namely, the euphemism of "letting nature take its course." There is (as we have seen) a long tradition in theology and moral philosophy of distinguishing between "letting die" and active "killing." And Hauerwas admits that in one sort of case the distinction does make sense – namely, where treatment is withheld because the prognosis is so poor that such care only prolongs death. And it is, of course, a medical judgment as to when the prognosis is actually so bleak.[15] In many other cases, though, life-prolonging treatment is withheld not because we are certain the child will die anyway but because we are afraid he/she will live. And to refer to treatment-refusal or respirator-removal as "letting die" in such cases is, in Hauerwas's estimation, a truly "strained" use of the term. In the Johns Hopkins and Bloomington Baby Doe cases, for example, refusal of surgery meant not a refusal to prolong death but a decision *for* certain death. And while we may choose to restrict our focus (and our language) to the physical distinction between acting and refraining from acting, the real question is "what is the proper description of the overall act" ([10], pp. 178–79). Hauerwas suggests that the proper description is "murder," and asks whether an injected air bubble might not have been more humane for all concerned. Indeed, he maintains that we would be "more moral" if we honestly face the fact that such choices constitute putting the child to death: "The murderer is more humane who does not live under the illusion that he is letting nature take its course for the good of humanity" ([4], p. 185; [10], pp. 178–80).

Of course, he notes, we all have our reasons for wanting to cling to the distinction between killing and letting die. Parents cannot bear to envision themselves as their children's executioners. And the physician, who "knows well" that refraining to give care means putting the child to death, nevertheless refuses to describe it as such because "as a doctor he fears the implications such a description might have for the care of future patients."[16] But both sorts of reasons are illusory and self-deceptive. Actually, Hauerwas suspects that the distinction is really a misleading way of gesturing our subtle shift toward seeing defective children as *strangers*. For we commonly admit that we have positive duties of aid toward our children, but we hold that our basic obligations toward strangers are largely negative – i.e., duties of noninterference. And our language of "refraining" to give aggressive medical treatment to defective neonates is really more the grammar of noninterference than of parental aid ([10], p. 179).

Having introduced and developed these interconnected lines of argument, Hauerwas offers, as a summary "framework within which ethical reflection must proceed," three general suggestions about neonatal care decisions ([10], p. 183). First, the "fundamental issue" providing the background for the amount and kind of care defective newborns should receive "is the obligations of parents to care for their children." This sounds rather obvious since, as he says, we "naturally want" to care for children. But defective babies challenge us to articulate our "natural" assumptions, since whether we should "normally" expect parental/medical aid under all conditions is not at all clear. Second, Hauerwas insists that parental care at least should not be determined by the extent of the child's "defect," unless that defect "is so physiologically severe that there is no potential for the child ever to benefit or respond to human care."[17] And, third, Hauerwas is not at all certain that the state should intervene legally to embody parental obligation in defective newborn cases. For, although the state has an interest in requiring parents to meet their basic obligations to their children, "it is a matter of debate whether such care is a 'basic' obligation." Instead, he offers the interesting recommendation that,

... [A]t the least ... each hospital and doctor [should] begin to draw up a statement of procedures concerning the care of defective newborns. This should be given to couples as early as possible so they might have an opportunity to find other institutions or doctors whose policies conform more exactly with their own ([10], p. 183).

Now, if we attempt to read these suggestions as policy recommendations, they appear to emphasize decisional procedure (i.e., *who* decides) as opposed to specific, criteria-bound decisional content – particularly when compared with, say, Ramsey's "medical indications policy." This is, of course, quite consistent with Hauerwas's emphasis upon *parental* care as the fundamental issue. But we must also remember that he does not consider parental responsibility as primarily a matter or "powers" or decisional "rights" in the first place; rather, it is an expression or embodiment of the *community's* narrative-based understanding of truth, humanity, and the good of children. So, he is willing to allow that societies such as ours also need to develop some "rules of thumb" to check our (parental) arbitrariness in difficult cases, and that such rules must be developed with the kind of "exactness" entailed by such cases rather than a generality which is open to perversion by our self-deception and self-justification. For, without social rules "all moral discourse becomes but a shadow play for deeper games of arbitrary power and of one man's domination of another" ([9], p. 233).

Even so, Hauerwas yet insists (with specific reference to any proposed criteria of 'humanhood' as a basis for treatment decisions) that "slavish dependence" on 'criteria,' 'rules of thumb,' etc., is not morally healthy:

I suspect that we are human exactly to the extent we can reach out and provide care for those who have no 'right' to it. Put more concretely, as important as criteria are to inform decisions, we cannot make them do all the work of ethical judgment and argument for all cases, since no criterion is going to relieve or should make less troublesome the burden of deciding to operate to save the life of a severely retarded child. To try to substitute 'impersonal criteria' for what should be the moral agony of such decisions is already to sacrifice more of our humanity than we can stand ([10], p. 162).

In other words, particular rules or criteria for neonatal treatment cannot in themselves illumine for us the moral reality of those situations. What we must have first is clear moral vision; and that is dependent on a community's truthful narrative, a story that makes sense of our lives and trains us to see clearly the moral meanings of human relationships and of 'care' in the face of finitude and tragedy.

4. FAMILY, COMMUNITY, AND MEDICAL EXPERIMENTATION WITH CHILDREN

Unlike McCormick and Ramsey, Hauerwas has not engaged in extensive published debate about the morality of nontherapeutic pediatric experimentation. But when the National Commission for the Protection of Human Subjects of

Biomedical and Behavioral Research was studying that issue in the mid-1970's, he was invited to submit an essay outlining his views (and responding to those of two other commentators). So the main lines of his argument as presented here are drawn primarily from that work ([8]; [16], pp. 125–41). As we will see, his reflections build largely upon themes already introduced in this chapter – the moral impoverishment of rights-based liberal ideology (as a foundation for medical or research practice), and familial and communitarian understandings of the meaning of 'child.'

To begin with, while much contemporary moral discussion of medical research tends to assume a general framework within which the 'rights' or interests of research subjects are contrasted with the interests or needs of larger populations of present and future sick persons, Hauerwas considers this a fundamentally mistaken and impoverished framework for moral reflection. He cites with approval Alasdair MacIntyre's lament that modern man's "central preoccupation" has become the prevention of interference with each other as we go about our own individual concerns ([26], pp. 22–23, cited in [16], p. 116). While the "classical" world view begins with the community of the *polis* and treats individual moral identity only within communities of citizenship and kinship, the "modern" view begins with the notion of a collection of individuals out of which social situations must somehow be constructed. One interesting result of the "modern" view, Hauerwas observes, is that the apparently antagonistic arguments of 'consequentialists' (for the greater good of the greater number) and 'deontologists' (for the inviolable rights of personal 'autonomy') may both actually share the same presuppositions of atomistic individualism. And both miss the real issue, namely, "what kind of risks should we as citizens and recipients of the benefits of health science be willing to undergo to further the general well-being of our community" ([16], p. 117).

Indeed, Hauerwas is critical of Ramsey on just this point. For, while Ramsey appeals to a Jewish/Christian notion of "covenant" (as well as Kant's notion of "respect for persons") to provide a model for his "canon of loyalty" in medical experimentation, it is not at all clear to Hauerwas how the analogy between God's covenant with his people and the doctor-patient canon of loyalty is either illuminating or justifiable. And the Kantian sense of "respect for persons" certainly seems too individualistic for any expression of the very *communitarian* conception of "covenant." To be a member of a covenant "is to be loyal to the commitments of a community in a manner that renders suspect the placing of individual interests before those of the community and the object of loyalty that the community serves" ([16], p. 134). Thus, Ramsey's argument is so weighed down with individualistic assumptions about how "no man is good enough to experiment upon another without his consent" that he avoids asking about "what ends medicine and collateral research ought to serve" ([16], p. 122).

Hauerwas frames this critique even more strikingly in *The Peaceable Kingdom* [13] where he suggests that our individualistic assumptions hide from us the truth that some members of our community must be subject to risks, and even suffering, if our community is to care about anything at all. For we are "necessarily tied together in a manner that mutually limits our lives." There is in fact *no* morality, he writes,

> ... that does not require others to suffer for our commitments. But there is nothing wrong with asking others to share and sacrifice for what we believe to be worthy. A more appropriate concern is whether what we commit ourselves to is worthy or not ([13], p. 9).

A "good society," then, cannot appeal solely to individual rights or strict policies of "informed consent"[18] in medical research or anything else. For, no *real* "society" can *exist* "when its citizens' only way of relating is in terms of noninterference" ([16], p. 130). Hauerwas does not reject all use of rights-language; he simply finds it insufficient as a basic moral language on grounds of social theory.

His criticism of rights-language is particularly acute when the issue at hand is the 'rights' of children. He admits that the notion of rights in childhood must seem to us to imply the sort of protection we think children should have. But such a notion is doubtful at best. In the first place, any attribution of 'rights' presupposes a moral psychology which, practically speaking, cannot be met by young children ([16], p. 130). More importantly, however, our attempts to employ rights-language with respect to children also imply that children are just one 'interest group' among others, and that we must establish procedural safeguards to protect their interests from incursion by other interest groups, including their parents ([16], p. 125). Put bluntly, rights-language manifests an attempt to give children some of the *power* their parents have. But that is "a formula for the destruction of the child" by trying to turn the child into an adult ([16], p. 132). Children need love, trust, and care – and none of these needs can be filled by giving them rights.

Morally, then, the question is not what rights-claims our children may have on us; it is rather what our responsibility toward them is, irrespective of their ability to make claims. And Hauerwas suggests that the reason why so many have tried to posit children's rights is because we need somehow to make up for the breakdown of our shared beliefs about the meaning of parental care for children ([16], p. 126). What we have overlooked, however, is that rights-theories are *needed* only when we assume that citizens "fundamentally relate to one another as strangers, if not outright enemies."[19] And to see the *family* as a contractual society of individuals is to see it as something it is not. Hauerwas prefers instead Aristotle's language of the family as a "natural" institution, at least in the sense that the family is a primitive institution prior to others (e.g, the State) and is not organized simply to satisfy basic desires. "In a decisive sense the family is not a voluntary institution and the kind of responsibilities that accrue in it are thus different" ([16], p. 128).

Indeed, the very meaning of 'child' is necessarily dependent upon some normative understanding of the meaning of 'family.' For, 'child' and 'children' denote moral roles relative to a set of practices and expectations we call 'family.' Children and their parents have duties toward one another, duties grounded in the concrete expectations of particular communities ([16], pp. 128–29). The primary responsibility of parents is to "initiate their children into the best form of life they know."[20] And the best form of life they know should not be seen as a matter of arbitrary, individualistic whim, but as something imparted through the existence and expectations of their community. So, to be a parent is to "perform an office for a community of seeing that a child finds his or her way to the moral best that the community has to offer." It may be argued, of course, that sometimes parents do not *know* what is best for their children, or that many children are quite capable of making sensible decisions for themselves. But these arguments are, in Hauerwas's view, "beside the point." The point is that in matters of importance parents *should know* what is best for their children. Moreover, children simply do not *have* important 'interests' until they have been taught what interests to have ([16], p. 133).

These reflections lead Hauerwas to offer partial approval of a notion of proxy consent for (nontherapeutic) pediatric experimentation. He rejects as "confused" the idea that proxy consent can and does protect the child's best interests (considered in isolation). But he suggests that it can be seen as an attempt to protect the *family unit's* integrity – at least where there is some shared community understanding of what purposes form the family's interests. In other words, proxy consent as an institution "is one way to insure that whatever is done to the child is done in accordance with the moral convictions and traditions of that family."[21] (Of course, he writes, the problem we see now, in our rights-based society, is that proxy consent has become simply a power in the hands of some parents whose moral convictions about care we find corrupt.)

Now, this understanding of proxy consent's meaning is also the basis for Hauerwas's criticism of one other (limited) defense of proxy consent we have already examined – that of Richard McCormick. Recall that McCormick approves of proxy consent in non-risky, high-benefit nontherapeutic research when we have reason to believe the child would consent, if capable, because he/she *ought* to consent. Hauerwas's problem with this is not that it imputes an unwarranted agency to children; indeed, he suspects that "children, even infants, can have a moral role in a community even before they are agents" ([16], p. 136). Rather, he is critical of McCormick's assumptions about how we *know* what a child "ought to want." For, McCormick's epistemic category (the universal natural law) is presented as offering us clear insight into what interests, or 'goods,' all persons should pursue. But, Hauerwas insists, there is really

> ... no way to determine what interests the child should have as a member of the human community *qua* human community. As humans we share a moral capacity and needs, but such capacity and needs are not sufficient to ground concrete moral judgements; that requires the convictions and practices of specific actual communities ([16], p. 137).

In the issue at hand, then, if a community's "primary purposes" are commonly seen to include a crucial role for medical research, then it may make sense to assume that everyone – including children – has an interest in research participation.

What Hauerwas suggests, however, is that such an assumption cannot be sustained *now*, in our society. We do not seem to have any shared commitments to medical research, and our apparent commitment to the ethics of noninterference with one another would seem to make any such societal consensus unlikely in the near future. Yet such a consensus is necessary before we can rise above simply arguing about the elements (and possibility) of informed consent. Thus, for instance, in arguing against those who would flatly forbid prisoners' and poor peoples' research participation because their consent is not fully 'uncoerced,' Hauerwas insists that such persons should not be denied the opportunity to "participate in the joint venture of our community to better our condition." But he finally ends up agreeing that their participation cannot be justified *until* medical experimentation "is seen as an opportunity – and perhaps even an obligation – for *everyone*" ([16], p. 120 – emphasis added).

This is perhaps our best clue as to what concrete public policy Hauerwas would favor with respect to nontherapeutic pediatric experimentation. For, in his comments to the National Commission he indicated that he was writing as if "an ideal world" of shared assumptions were possible; and he admitted that he frankly did not know what kind of policy he would recommend if he were on the Commission. Instead, he concluded his remarks – and I will conclude this section – with three general suggestions ([16], pp. 140–41). First, if we are to experiment on children at all, we should do so "very, very carefully." Second, a "more radical" suggestion would be that, since we presently seem to have no moral clarity as to the meaning or shared goals of experimentation, perhaps we should not use children in nontherapeutic research at all. Or, finally,

> ... it might be interesting to say only the broadest guidelines can be drawn and that the justification of each experiment depends greatly on how the experiments can morally articulate their purpose as a way to serve particular people (the health of the nation will not do) and why the children and parents of the experiment have a stake in that purpose ... Protocols, like judicial decisions, should have moral dicta which show us how they are justified in the light of our basic convictions.

Once again, then, we see that Hauerwas's theological-ethical approach cannot be constrained by the language (or reasoning) of an ethic of consequences, nor of an ethic of abstract principles and derived rules. Instead, he articulates an ethic of character, both personal and communitarian. Such character requires moral vision and imagination so that we can recognize and assimilate ourselves into those narratives that give coherence and meaning to our lives. No 'situation' we face is isolable; we must develop the skills necessary to 'fit' the events and choices we face into the story we live. Moreover, our individual life-narratives are not isolable, either; we cannot create our own life stories *de novo*. Rather, we are formed by the narratives of our communities just as we propagate those stories ourselves by living them.

This understanding of moral life emphasizes in great degree our imaginative powers of *description*. For those powers are essential in answering the questions, "What sort of persons are we?" and "What, in truth, is going on here?" – questions which are prior to any question of what we should *do*. Only when we can describe truthfully ourselves and our existence can we recognize those commitments which guide our recognition of, and response in, situations of moral choice.

NOTES

[1] [5], p. 102. Hauerwas expresses sympathy with G.H. Mead's conception of the social self, but is critical of Mead's social determinism and tendency to reduce the agential "I" to the social "me." Our current problem, as Hauerwas sees it, is that our modern pluralist society is providing an enormous multiplicity of available descriptions through which persons form themselves; thus their 'freedom' is stressed, but the assumption of *who we are* has become more problematic in such a differentiated society. (See [5], p. 103 fn.)

[2] See Hauerwas's discussion of Murdoch's arguments in [4], Chapter 2.

[3] At one point Hauerwas cites with approval Jean Giraudoux' definition of 'tragedy' as "... the affirmation of a horrible bond between men and a greater fate than man's fate" ([10], p. 12).

[4] Hauerwas's many references to the Christian story's message of non-violence relate primarily to physical (e.g., military) expressions of violence, although at times he seems to include under the umbrella of 'violence' all manipulative or coercive attempts at pursuation of others (as expressions of one's own will-to-power). However, his writings display relatively little analysis of what the Christian story has to say about the 'violence' of economic and psycho-social oppression and exclusion perpetuated by contemporary political, social and economic structures (including the Church itself). Gloria Albrecht has argued that, while Hauerwas rightly rejects liberalism's confidence in ahistorical human reason as a source of universal truth, he effectively replaces it with a "fixed Christian narrative" *as seen from within his own particular social location* and which functions in the same universalizing manner, masking important differences that emerge when the Christian story is viewed from other locations in the Christian community. As a result, Hauerwas tends to 'see' the moral issue of violence (and other moral issues) only from a position that is already relatively comfortable, privileged, and "in control." But, Albrecht writes, when an analysis of social location is applied to Hauerwas claims, then

... the social source of [his] ethics of character becomes clear. The social loyalties of [his] theological anthropology are exposed and the material consequences revealed. The violence of continual participation in unjust social structures is called non-violence. Participating with others in the risk of complex, often ambiguous and limited acts toward creating and embodying social structures of justice is condemned as participation in the unfaithful and violent desire to control history. Renouncing efforts to transform the unjust power relations that benefit the white, middle- and upper-classes is honored as "losing control." Choosing to act in ways which challenge such power is denounced as will-to-power ([1], Chapter 4).

And it must be noted that Hauerwas tends to *invite* this kind of criticism when he offers such comments as, ". . . the current fashion to identify with the 'oppressed,' admirable though it may be, lacks moral intelligibility. We end up in the shabby game of trying to figure out who is the most oppressed" ([22], p. 3).

[5] Just as he claims to know that the Christian story has been inherently pacifist all along, Hauerwas also claims to know how the Church has "always" felt about abortion. Yet, his historical and theological interpretations relating to the latter issue have not gone unchallenged (see [3], for example).

[6] See, for example, his chapter (with David Burrell) in [10] entitled "Self-Deception and Autobiography: Reflections on Speer's *Inside the Third Reich*," which describes how Albert Speer's lack of assimilation into a truthful narrative left him without the skills necessary to recognize or challenge the "demonic" story of Hitler's National Socialism.

[7] [5], p. 114. Put differently, "free will" does not describe a *faculty* of the self, but "the way we decide to engage in actions under certain descriptions rather than others" ([4], p. 65).

[8] [10], p. 115. In a footnote, Hauerwas and Bondi express approval of Ramsey's (penultimate) policy of (1) medical indications, and (2) the dying patient's wishes (p. 230, n. 35). However, Hauerwas later seems to deny Ramsey's 'medicalization' of the *determination* of when "the dying process" begins (see [16], pp. 33, 106).

[9] Hauerwas is usually critical of any moral distinction between killing and letting die. (This issue will be addressed in the next section.)

[10] He does, however, aver in *Suffering Presence* that Robert Veatch is correct in his suggestion that "a right to refuse treatment" is a better means of considering the euthanasia question than the traditional ordinary/extraordinary means distinction ([16], p. 93).

[11] [10], p. 177. Hauerwas broadens the same point to rebut utilitarian arguments for letting a few expensively-treated babies die in order to afford relief of suffering for many others; for such is "a charity run wild and gone crazy" because it *cannot* relieve the world of all its suffering ([4], p. 193).

[12] [10], p. 167. This particular point has an uncharacteristically utilitarian ring to it. It is presented, though, as one 'point to consider' among many others, and does not carry the weight of Hauerwas's overall argument.

[13] Likewise, to be a "man" is to be able to "perceive and respond to other men with recognition of care" ([10], p. 162).

[14] See Chapter 1.

[15] [10], p. 178. Hauerwas's approval of 'letting die' in such circumstances looks very much like Ramsey's criterion of "medically contraindicated" treatment (see Chapter 3). However, as we have seen, Hauerwas does not follow Ramsey's insistence that medical indications should be determinative in choosing or rejecting *one's own* life-prolonging treatment.

[16] [10], p. 166. Hauerwas admits that this may be a "good moral reason" to maintain the distinction, in order to "enforce the doctor's commitment to save life." Even so, it is then important that we develop criteria for careful application of the distinction.

[17] Hauerwas also adds, in *Vision and Virtue* ([4], p. 185), that treatment decisions for (any) dying patients "must be based solely on considerations of [their] welfare," and not on considerations of society or family benefits.

[18] Hauerwas also notes that genuinely informed consent is widely believed to be impossible to obtain; and even if it were possible, there are yet "some things we should not do to ourselves even for the good of others" ([16], p. 119).

[19] [16], p. 128. Of course, the defender of liberal rights-theories might object at this point that Hauerwas seems to have read a great deal of Hobbesian social contract theory and not much Locke or Rousseau!

[20] [16], p. 132. Hauerwas also defines the "goal" of parenting as "the creation of people who can enter into trustful relations because they have learned not to fear the other as a threat to their 'autonomy.'"

[21] [16], p. 135. Moreover, as we saw in the previous section, Hauerwas believes it is best to see the physician's obligations of care to the child as "an extension of the *parent's* basic responsibilities." Any 'claim' the child would have on the physician is "mediated through the responsibilities of the parents" ([16], p. 139).

REFERENCES

1. Albrecht, G.: 1992, 'Myself and Other Characters: A Feminist Response to Hauerwas's Ethics of Character', unpublished Ph.D. dissertation, Temple University (publication forthcoming from Abingdon Press as *The Chracter of Our Communities*).
2. Gustafson, J.: 1985, 'The Sectarian Temptation: Reflections on Theology, the Church, and the University', *Proceedings of the Catholic Theological Society* 40, 83–94.
3. Harrison, B.: 1983, *Our Right to Choose: Toward a New Ethic of Abortion*, Beacon Press, Boston.
4. Hauerwas, S.: 1974, *Vision and Virtue: Essays in Christian Ethical Reflection*, University of Notre Dame Press, Notre Dame.
5. Hauerwas, S.: 1975, *Character and the Christian Life: A Study in Theological Ethics*, Trinity University Press, San Antonio, Texas.
6. Hauerwas, S.: 1975, 'The Ethicist as Theologian', *The Christian Century*, April 24, p. 409.
7. Hauerwas, S.: 1977, 'Learning to See Red Wheelbarrows: On Vision and Relativism', *Journal of the American Academy of Religion* 45/2 (Supplement, June), 643–55.
8. Hauerwas, S.: 1977, 'Rights, Duties, and Experimentation on Children: A Critical Response to Worsford and Bartholome', *Research Involving Children: APPENDIX* (National Commission for the Protection of Human Subjects of Biomedical and Behavioral Research, DHEW Publication No. [OS] 77–0005), Washington, D.C. (Edited and republished in [16], pp. 125–41.)
9. Hauerwas, S.: 1977, 'Selecting Children to Live or Die: An Ethical Analysis of the Debate Between Dr. Lorber and Dr. Freeman on the Treatment of Meningomyelocele', in D. Horan and D. Mall (eds.), *Death, Dying, and Euthanasia*, University Publications of America, Washington, D.C., pp. 228–49.
10. Hauerwas, S.: 1977, *Truthfulness and Tragedy: Further Investigations Into Christian Ethics*, Fides Press, Notre Dame.
11. Hauerwas, S.: 1978, 'Can Ethics Be Theological?' (Review of J. Gustafson, *Protestant and Roman Catholic Ethics*, and P. Ramsey, *Ethics at the Edges of Life*), *Hastings Center Report* 8/5, pp. 47–49.
12. Hauerwas, S.: 1981, *A Community of Character: Toward a Constructive Christian Social Ethic*, University of Notre Dame Press, Notre Dame.
13. Hauerwas, S.: 1983, *The Peaceable Kingdom: A Primer in Christian Ethics*, University of Notre Dame Press, Notre Dame.
14. Hauerwas, S.: 1985, *Against the Nations: War and Survival in a Liberal Society*, Winston-Seabury Press, Minneapolis.

15. Hauerwas, S.: 1985, 'On Medicine and Virtue: A Response', in E. Shelp (ed.), *Virtue and Medicine*, D. Reidel, Dordrecht, Netherlands, pp. 347–55.
16. Hauerwas, S.: 1986, *Suffering Presence: Theological Reflections on Medicine, the Mentally Handicapped, and the Church*, University of Notre Dame Press, Notre Dame.
17. Hauerwas, S.: 1988, *Christian Existence Today: Essays on Church, World, and Living In Between*, Labyrinth Press, Durham, N.C.
18. Hauerwas, S.: 1990, *Naming the Silences: God, Medicine, and the Problem of Suffering*, Eerdmans, Grand Rapids.
19. Hauerwas, S.: 1991, *After Christendom? How the Church is to Behave if Freedom, Justice, and a Christian Nation are Bad Ideas*, Abingdon, Nashville.
20. Hauerwas, S.: 1993, *Unleashing the Scripture: Freeing the Bible from Captivity to America*, Abingdon, Nashville.
21. Hauerwas, S.: 1993, 'Why I am Neither a Communitarian nor a Medical Ethicist', *Hastings Center Report* 23/6, S9–S10.
22. Hauerwas, S.: 1994, *Dispatches from the Front: Theological Engagements with the Secular*, Duke University Press, Durham.
23. Hauerwas, S. and Willimon, W.: 1985, 'Embarrassed by God's Presence', *The Christian Century*, Jan. 30, 98–100
24. Hauerwas, S. and Willimon, W.: 1989, *Resident Aliens: Life in the Christian Colony*, Abingdon, Nashville.
25. Lammers, S.: 1993, 'On Stanley Hauerwas: Theology, Medical Ethics, and the Church', in A. Verhey and S. Lammers (eds.), *Theological Voices in Medical Ethics*, Eerdmans, Grand Rapids, pp. 57–77.
26. MacIntyre, A.: 1978, 'How to Identify Ethical Principles', in *The Belmont Report* (DHEW Publication No. [OS] 78–0013), Washington, D.C., pp. 22–33.
27. Marty, M.: 1989, 'Impolite Disenglobments', *The Christian Century* 106 (May 3), p. 487.
28. Ogletree, T.: 1980, 'Character and Narrative: Stanley Hauerwas' Studies of the Christian Life', *Religious Studies Review* 6/1, 25–30.
29. Outka, G.: 1980, 'Character, Vision and Narrative', *Religious Studies Review* 6/2, 110–18.

CHAPTER FIVE

JAMES GUSTAFSON: PIETY AND THE ETHICS OF THEOCENTRIC DISCERNMENT

One of the points of comparison raised in this study is the extent to which each moralist's work depends upon theological insights or beliefs in making moral claims – or, in other words, the extent to which each considers his applied ethics to be "distinctively Christian." We have seen genuine variety, both in their views about theological sources for moral knowledge and in their assessments of which theological themes or concepts should be central to our understanding of moral life.

The final figure to be examined here, James Gustafson, has been an ardent and frequent critic of those "religious ethicists" trained in theology who nevertheless reflect upon medical-ethical issues in ways which do not reflect explicitly their own religious convictions or theological traditions. Of such "common denominator" ethics he wrote, in 1978, that,

> ... [M]uch theological or 'religious' writing is directed to the justification of an enterprise in the eyes of persons who are not really interested enough to care whether the justification is adequate or not. (I worked for years on a book *Can Ethics Be Christian?* with the nagging sense that most persons who answer in an unambiguous affirmative would not be interested in my supporting argument, that a few fellow professional persons might be interested enough to look at it, and that for those who believe the answer is negative the question itself is not sufficiently important to bother about.) While theologians ought to continue to participate competently in the public debates about matters of technology and the life sciences, they would also do well to attend to the home folks who *might* care more about what they have to say ...
>
> It is the 'religious ethicists' who have most to be anxious about, in my judgment. They will have either to become moral philosophers with a special interest in 'religious' texts and arguments, or become theologians: Christian theologians, or natural theologians, or 'religious dimensions' theologians. Only indifference to what they are writing, or exceeding patience with inexcusable ambiguity, can account for the tolerance they have enjoyed ([11], p. 386).

The harshness of this judgment indicates the seriousness of Gustafson's concern that the role of religious ethicists should be to indicate clearly how "religion *qualifies* morality."[1] In his view, the task of ethical reflection flows, both in content and in method, from the task of theological reflection. He has summarized the major foci or themes of his own work by offering the following description of what it means to "say something theological": "To say something theological is to say something religious. Theology has its deepest significance within the context of *piety*, and in the context of a historic *religious tradition*. To say something theological is to say something about *how things really and ultimately are*. To say something theological is to say something *ethical*."[2] These themes and their interrelatedness are treated at length in Gustafson's most systematic study in theological ethics, the two-volume *Ethics From a Theocentric Perspective* ([14], [16]). In that work he seeks to establish a framework of assumptions and parameters within which theological inquiry legitimately can be conducted and theological claims made; then he describes the "perspective" appropriate to this mode of inquiry which allows us to "discern" divine intentionalities for purposes of moral being and doing.

Now, like the three other moralists examined here thus far, Gustafson appropriates selected themes and symbols from Scripture and tradition in formulating his theological proposal. Unlike them, however, he moves beyond a re-articulation of traditional Christian theological themes to a more foundational, experience-based model of discerning theological truths. In so doing, he finds that he must alter or even reject certain traditionally-accepted tenets of Christian faith. Thus, while he shares Hauerwas's strong insistence upon the 'qualification' of all theological ethics, his project does not share Hauerwas's emphasis on the necessity (for moral agency) of a community's formation through the particularity of its tradition's narratives. Indeed, Gustafson's approach involves, in the words of Gerald McKenny, "breaking down the barrier between universality and particularity" ([26], p. 512).

It is crucial, then, that we attend to the form and content of Gustafson's ethical theory by first attending to some of the specifics of his theological method. Most of the explication of his approach presented here (in the first two sections of this chapter) will be drawn from the *Ethics From a Theocentric Perspective*. Following that, the remaining three sections will examine implications of a "theocentric ethics" for issues of medical treatment refusal, neonatal care decisions, and nontherapeutic pediatric research.

1. THEOCENTRISM AND PIETY

To begin with, Gustafson defines "theology" primarily as an activity of the practical reason which involves reflection upon that particular dimension of the human experience denoted "religious." By "religious" he means that dimension of experience (not consciously shared by all) that "senses a relationship to an ultimate power that sustains and stands over against humans and the world" ([8], p. 4f.; [14], p. 158f.). This ultimate power is not experienced immediately and directly, but always indirectly and in a mediated way – in other words, always as, at the same time, an experience of something else ([8], p. 5f.). The discipline of theology, then, seeks to draw inferences from the religious dimension of experience about the ultimate power's qualities and characteristics, purposes and intentions, and relations to the world ([8], p. 7). It cannot be denied that theology (as a discipline) has deeply speculative aspects; but it also has a basically *practical* character, in that its inferences are testable according to their adequacy in providing meaning and coherence for life in the presence of a powerful Other, in the kind of direction for human action they offer, and in their congruence with inferences from a broad range of human experiences ([14], p. 158f.).

Like theology, "ethics" is also an activity of practical reason; it is a reflection on those dimensions of human experience denoted "moral." It seeks to "analyze the necessary conditions for moral activity" and to "indicate normatively what moral principles and values ought to govern human action" ([8], p. 13).

Now, religion *qualifies* moral experience when one chooses and acts not simply in response to other persons, events, and things, but also in response to the ultimate power sustaining and standing over against creation. Likewise, the "*theological* qualification of *ethics*" occurs through articulation of the ultimate power's significance "both as a necessary condition for moral action, and as a necessary justification for moral values and principles that judge, prescribe, and govern action" ([8], p. 13f.).

Having offered these generic definitions of his enterprise, Gustafson goes on to aver, at great length, that a major transformation is necessary in the dominant perspective of contemporary theological ethics: namely, a transformation from "anthropocentrism" to "theocentrism." In his view, the major strand of both religious and secular Western ethics has held that material considerations for morality should be derived from purely human points of reference; or, in other words, moral norms have been posited or accepted with solely human (individual and social) value or benefit as their focus. Man the *measurer* of all things has also been man the *measure* of all things; all things have been put into human service ([14], pp. 82, 88). Even those views of Christianity most focused upon divine governance have pointed to the human-centered benefits (e.g., peace or prosperity in earthly life, and 'eternal life' thereafter) for believers. This is nothing but "utilitarian religion" in Gustafson's estimation ([14], p. 16ff.).

In contrast to this, biblical morality had an objective, non-anthropocentric referent for material moral considerations: the will of God, not man ([14], p. 89). We have no good evidence from Scripture that human well-being (or salvation) is the central purpose or goal of the divine ordering and governance of things. Moreover, there is evidence from other aspects of human experience (especially the sciences) to rebut any view of humankind as the purposive 'crown' of creation:

From what we know about the development of our universe, the development of the preconditions for the evolution of life on our planet, the development of various species and the extinction of many, the contingencies ... that occurred which made possible the evolution of mammals, and the forecasts for the future demise of our universe (to be sure, in billions of years), it is very difficult to sustain the belief that the cosmos was made for man ([14], p. 90; see also p. 83).

Gustafson admits that some biblical writings do seem to have a pronounced God-for-man perspective (and that his own offering of biblical warrants for his interpretive proposal is selective), but he insists that there is plenty of evidence for his conviction that Christian theology has grossly exaggerated the place of humanity in the overall scheme of things. Indeed, it is this "egocentric predicament" which has created the problem of theodicy, since the theodicy question "arises only on the assumption that God necessarily wills the good of a particular person or community as that good is humanly understood" ([14], p. 96).

What can be said, then, of a theological ethics in which the Deity's will is not assumed to be coincident with what we consider to be "the good" from our own "anthropocentric" perspective? Well, Gustafson confesses that it may not look like "ethics" at all in the traditional sense of Christianity and Western culture. But he insists that theological ethics must be fundamentally *theocentric* if it is to recognize that only God is God, that only God establishes the place of humankind within the entire created order, and that only God is then the *measure* of all things. Thus, what is right for man "has to be determined in relation to man's place in the universe and, indeed, in relation to the will of God for all things as that might dimly be discerned" ([14], p. 99). The central question for theocentric ethics is, then, "what is God enabling and requiring us to be and to do?" And Gustafson's initial answer is that "we are to relate ourselves and all things in a manner appropriate to their relations to God" ([14], pp. 327, 113).

Of course, such a question and answer forces us back upon the prior question: How can we come to know, or at least infer, anything about God and the divine ordering of relations between God, ourselves, and all things in creation? Gustafson's answer to this is what makes this theological program such a profound challenge to much contemporary and traditional theology and ethics. Thus, it deserves our focused attention here.

To begin with, despite his cogent and impassioned critique of anthropocentrism, Gustafson points out that "a certain kind of anthropocentrism" is unavoidable in theological reflection. For, theology and ethics are but reflection upon prior religious and moral *experience*. All knowledge of God is *human* knowledge, mediated through human experience ([14], p. 115). Human beings are, unavoidably, the knowers and the measurers of what can be known through many sorts of experience. And human experiences are rarely individualistic; their explanations and meanings are defined, shared, and tested *socially*, in communities which share common objects of attention and interest, some common symbols, concepts, etc. ([14], pp. 120, 129). Further, experience-construing beliefs, symbols, and explanations are not only social but *historical*; their validity and adequacy are tested with reference to the most accurate body of 'facts' accepted by communities within their particular historical contexts. This means, among other things, that "any organized community that freezes its requirements for membership according to the symbols and explanations adequate at a particular time is bound to have difficulties, especially in the modern world" ([14], p. 124).

In addition to these preliminary convictions, Gustafson goes on to argue that religious (and moral) experience has profoundly *affective* as well as cognitive and volitional aspects. "Religion is, in an important way, a matter of affectivity" ([14], pp. 195, 119). There are, he writes, certain senses or sensibilities evoked within human experience of selves, objects, events (and especially within the experience of "others") on the basis of which we may draw theological inferences (that is, inferences about the divine "Other"). These religiously-significant senses are: *dependence*; *gratitude*; *obligation*; *remorse* and *repentance*; *possibility* (for altering oppressive conditions or sustaining ones which are supportive); and *direction* toward ends or goals ([14], pp. 129–34; see also [7], Chapter 4) Now, all of these senses are quite "natural" or even "ordinary" in human personal and social experience; they are construed in various ways by "radically secular" persons and communities as well as religious ones. The step which distinguishes the "religious" consciousness from the secular, however, occurs when what is sensed is the reality of the presence of "that which is beyond the means of scientific investigation and proof." In monotheistic religions, this step involves a move or leap from the experience of others (or of "otherness") to the senses of respect, reverence, dependence, gratitude, etc. toward "*an* Other" – toward that ultimate power which limits and sustains life in the world ([14], pp. 135, 195–97).

Gustafson hastens to point out that affectivity is not antithetical to or set over against intellect or reason. They are both integral to human experience and to reflection on it. Religion and morality are not simply matters of willing or doing what "reason" requires; nor are they matters of feelings and emotions alone. Rational perceptions can both evoke and limit our affective responses, just as affectivity – our attitudes, dispositions, and emotions – influence our motivations, perceptions, and "reasons" for responding ([14], p. 199f.).

But the trend in both theology and ethics, as Gustafson sees it, has been to minimize or discount the significance of affectivity in favor of cognitive or volitional explanations. (This has been especially apparent since the Enlightenment era, and is a particularly profound legacy of Kantian thought.) One result of this is a dilution of the meaning of *faith*, that most traditional hallmark notion of religious consciousness. For many people, faith is contrasted with reason, since the former is seen to refer to that knowledge accepted on some authority other than reason and experience. Also, faith is often seen to mean trust or confidence of a particular sort – namely, a confidence (unfounded, in Gustafson's view) that God's purposes are the fulfillment of my self-measured and self-chosen interests ([14], pp. 201–203).

For these reasons (and others) Gustafson argues that we should move our focus from the notion of "faith" to a more accurate focus on religious affectivity, and particularly to that most central religious affection: *piety*. Piety is a settled disposition or attitude toward the world and toward God, characterized most fundamentally by awe and respect (and not to be confused with "piousness" or sanctimoniousness). It certainly encompasses the notion of "faith" as a "measured confidence in God," but not as a confidence that God's purpose is to fulfill human purposes ([14], pp. 201, 203). Moreover, an understanding of piety in terms of awe and respect makes clear that our religious affections may include both an attraction and an aversion to the powers of God as we experience them – "both a love of God, the giver of the possibilities for value and meaning in life, and fear and anger in the face of conditions which frustrate human aspirations and threaten or deny human life" ([14], p. 204).

Now, as noted previously, piety and other religious affections are evoked by quite ordinary objects and events; we do not experience God as a distinct object, but only through other objects of experience. But senses (such as dependence, gratitude, etc.) can lead us to religious interpretation of their ultimate object. Generally, this move begins when we ask questions of great religious significance about our experiences. Gustafson cites four such questions: In whom or in what can we have confidence?; To whom or what do we owe loyalty?; For what can we, or ought we, to hope?; and What are the appropriate objects of human loves, desires, or aversions? ([14], p. 224f.). These questions can be and are asked within many arenas of presumptively non-religious experience (and Gustafson mentions five of these arenas: nature, history, culture, society, and self) ([14], pp. 207–23). Our answers to these questions delineate our "religion," in Gustafson's explication of the matter. (He points out, too, that many persons' answers do not lead to affirmation of any ultimate power's presence; thus he concludes that there are "functional surrogates to religion as I understand it" – [14], p. 225.)

This move to religious affectivity and explanation through asking and answering religiously significant questions is certainly a crucial step in Gustafson's model of theology's genesis. He is willing, too, to admit to a certain "circularity" in this process: my answers to these questions about my experience will confirm what I am predisposed to have them confirm ([14], p. 233f.). And that predisposition is rooted in two "subjective" factors: individual, creative formulation of religious ideas based upon convictions formed to inter-connect present with past experiences; and our "reliance upon a particular historical [religious] tradition, at least initially." In other words, religious affectivity grows not only from our integrative responses to putatively non-religious aspects of experience but also from being informed by "the constituting events, the significant persons, the history of the community, and the stories that are borne through time by the Christian tradition and by the churches" ([14], pp. 230–31). What Gustafson wants to stress, however, is that one is not merely a product of his/her tradition's "socialization"; the tradition's symbols become personally meaningful in a world-construing way when one *consents* to them. Consent is not "resignation" but rather a matter of being persuaded that the tradition's symbols are adequate, reasonable and meaningful in interpreting our experience of the created world ([14], p. 232). When traditional symbols are no longer evocative and meaningful for experience-construing persons and communities, then they give way to new or altered symbols which are adequate.

To summarize part of what has been said thus far, Gustafson asserts that theology must begin with the reality of human *experience*. Our responses to experiences integrate *affective* as well as cognitive and volitional aspects of our selves; thus our responses often take the form of "senses," attitudes or dispositions. When our experiences evoke responses which involve questions about ultimate powers bearing down on us and sustaining us through those experiences, then the affectivities involved are of a "religious" sort; the primary religious affection is *piety*, manifest characteristically in awe and reverence for the ultimate power. The "answers" we affirm, in response to our questions about ultimate power and significance, are formulated in light of their coherence with our own construal of the world we experience and also in light of the interpretive symbols of the traditions we inherit. Both persons and traditional communities of persons must continually test inherited symbols for their adequacy and coherence in construing our relations to God and the world – especially their coherence with other claims we can make from other aspects of human knowledge and experience, broadly conceived.

In light of this description of the genesis of religious ideas, Gustafson makes two fundamental claims about the theological enterprise. The first is that piety (rather than "belief") is a "necessary condition for ideas of God to be subjectively meaningful and intellectually persuasive" ([14], p. 257). The second – and more controversial – claim is that religious symbols and ideas are not valid if they do not comport with what we know from the physical and social sciences. Following Ernst Troeltsch, Gustafson insists that,

The substantial content of theology, if it is not in perfect harmony with scientific knowledge, cannot be in sharp incongruity with it, and what we say about God must be congruent in some way with what we know about human experience and its objects through the sciences ([14], p. 251f.).

These two claims form a general basis for 'testing' the adequacy of traditional assertions about God and God's relations to humanity and the world. In Gustafson's assessment of historical religious traditions, it is (parts of) the Reformed tradition which can be justified most fully on the grounds he has set forth. He points to three principal themes of Reformed theology which are most properly stressed: (1) a sense of a powerful, sovereign Other; (2) the centrality of piety in religious and moral life; and (3) an understanding that all human activity should be ordered properly according to what can be discerned about God's purposes ([14], pp. 163f., 195). Given these themes, he goes on to note that certain "classic" theological symbols can be sustained as viable ways of speaking about God's relation to humanity and the world – those of God as Creator, as Sustainer and Governor of the "ordering" of creation, as Judge, and as Redeemer ([14], pp. 236–51).

Applying his test of scientific congruence to these traditional themes and symbols, Gustafson offers several substantive conclusions about *what* we can discern of God's purposes. First, "many of the data and theories of many sciences" support the religious sense of *dependence* upon powers beyond ourselves. We experience a substantial dependence upon both natural and cultural processes. Both the limits and the possibilities for personal and communal flourishing are shaped by powers outside ourselves. Second, there is also scientific evidence for an "*ordering*" of natural developments and processes. (Gustafson avoids using "order" as a noun because of its suggestion of a static, immutable, trans-temporal and trans-cultural "order of nature" – as in much traditional natural law theory, which he finds indefensible on the evidence.) The most one can say of the natural ordering is that "a 'governance' is occurring"; it does not offer sufficient warrant for belief in a "designer" or in any "final purposiveness" in nature ([14], pp. 261–62).

Third, the clear presence of ordering in the realms of history, culture, and society can offer inferences about the fundamental requisites for humanity's survival. Piety can discern the presence of an ordering power which creates conditions of *possibility* for creativity and initiative, for personal development, scientific and artistic achievements, the development of institutions, etc. There is, too, a perception of proper ordering in the *moral* realm, inasmuch as "certain fundamental requisites must be met in some way for human life to flourish properly." Piety construes this as a discernment of the ultimate power's moral governance ([14], pp. 263–64).

Finally, the sciences can contribute substantively to theology by indicating "certain *directions* that the empowerment and ordering of life takes, and with which human beings must cooperate." We must pay attention to the "direction" of personal, natural, cultural and historical ordering not just for the sake of our own flourishing but for the sake of "the natural world itself" ([14], p. 264).

In addition to these general congruences between piety's construal and the evidences of science, Gustafson also offers important examples of theological inferences that are *not* plausible in piety and in view of scientific knowledge. We have no evidence, for instance, that humanity is the culmination and *telos* of creation. To those who would offer the theory of evolution as evidence of such a view, he responds that if there were a divine plan (with divine "foreknowledge") in bringing the evolutionary process to fruition in human life, "there was no particular merit in bringing it into being through such an inefficient and lengthy process." Moreover, it is scientifically evident that "as the beginning was without us, so will the end also be without us."

The Apocalypse and other traditional Christian eschatological symbols are not scientifically supportable and therefore must be questioned ([14], pp. 267–68). And, as we noted earlier, theocentric piety – and certainly the sciences – neither require nor offer plausible evidence for any notion of "eternal life" or "resurrection destiny" ([14], pp. 183–84).

As for other, particular attributes of divine powers, Gustafson warns that we should avoid not only anthropocentrism but also anthropomorphism in our construal:

> It is my conviction that if we choose to use the analogy of agency for construing the Deity, it must be developed with great circumspection. Insofar as the analogy leads us to assert that God has intelligence, like but superior to our own, and that God has a will, a capacity to control events comparable to the more radical claims made for human beings, the claims are excessive ([14], p. 270).

While we can discern divine *purposes* through human experience and knowledge of life in the world, Gustafson holds (with Tillich) that we can be personally related to those purposes without conceiving God in anthropomorphic terms. Moreover, we can (and should) understand those purposes as "good" *without* claiming that they are good *for us*, individually or collectively. It seems clear, for instance, that the divine governance expressed through nature is "not necessarily beneficent" from a human point of view. Indeed, piety evoked in us in the presence of divine powers "can be expressed in fear as well as gratitude" ([14], p. 272). For, piety infers the truth: that the purposes of divine governance are "not all directed toward us." Further, discernment of processes of divine governance in the world does not sustain any inference of rigid divine *determinism*. While we are led to acknowledge the many continuities between human beings and other things in nature, and the conditions which both limit and sustain our possibilities for action, experience shows us that we are yet able to respond to the divine governance by responding to persons and events in an "interactive" way. Our choices and actions are *responses*, yes, but they are not simply the "effects of describable and knowable sufficient causes" ([14], pp. 273–74).

Now, before we depart from this account of what Gustafson believes we can (and cannot) validly infer about God in relation to humanity and the world, we should also take note of the Christology that emerges from his theocentric proposal. For, he has been accused of presenting a theology which is not recognizably Christian.[3] And while Gustafson himself claims that Christology is "the most critical doctrinal issue" for any Christian theology, he also insists that his goal has not been to defend traditional Christianity but rather to "find what can be most truly claimed about God" ([14], pp. 275, 279).

So, then, what can be most truly claimed about Jesus? Gustafson's assertions, he says, are derived primarily from the narratives of the synoptic gospels. He explains his selective appeal to Scripture on the basis of his

PIETY AND THE ETHICS OF THEOCENTRIC DISCERNMENT 139

sense that narrative has priority over more "abstract" language in evoking and sustaining piety, but also because he rejects "biblicistic views of revelation" and because of his "epistemological suspicion" of the meaningfulness of Christological claims (e.g., about the "preexistent Christ") in the epistolary theologies ([14], p. 275, n. 65). These explanations make it rather clear that he parts company with those who advocate so-called "high" Christologies. Instead, Gustafson wants to argue that "Jesus incarnates theocentric piety and fidelity." The gospel narratives of his life and ministry allow us to "see and know something of the powers that bear down on us and sustain us, and of the piety and the manner of life that are appropriate to them." Jesus's life, ministry and teachings are an "historical embodiment" of what God is enabling and requiring us to be and to do. The Christian community is what it is through its consent to the power of the gospels to inform us about the purposes of the divine governance, just as the primitive church saw Jesus as the Christ through its consent to his powers. Indeed, "the only good reason for claiming to be Christian is that we continue to be empowered, sustained, renewed, informed, and judged by Jesus's incarnation of theocentric piety and fidelity" ([14], pp. 276–77).

While Gustafson refers at one point to "the powers of Jesus," he does not mention what those powers might be, other than the exemplary (and thus evocative) power of Jesus's witness. And it is perhaps instructive that the one basis he cites for our capacity to find "insight into the correctness of a theocentric vision" in the gospel narratives is that the "fundamental human experiences" they describe are similar to those of our surroundings ([14], p. 277).

In sum, Gustafson seems to reject metaphysical or transcendental claims about Jesus as the Christ in favor of claims about Jesus's truly theocentric construal of shared human experiences of the divine governance. Jesus's evocative power for us appears to rest in the gospels' assertions *that* he construed things *as* he did. Those of us looking on from more 'traditional' theological perspectives are yet left with many Christological questions – for instance, the question of whether Gustafson's Jesus is 'unique' in any sense other than the *degree* of his theocentric piety. At any rate, while Gustafson may insist that Christology is a "critical doctrinal issue" for his proposal, it does not appear that his theological method, or even most of his substantive conclusions, stands or falls on any of his Christological claims.

The purpose of this section has been to illustrate the various facets, both traditional and novel, of Gustafson's theological method. In particular, we have sought to trace his developmental moves from immediate objects of human experience to a perspective of theocentric piety in which substantive claims about divine ordering and governance can be inferred and tested. The next section will broaden this inquiry by focusing upon the moral expression of theocentric piety in our being and doing in the world.

2. THEOCENTRIC ETHICS: PARTICIPATION, DISCERNMENT, AND RELATING PARTS AND WHOLES

Earlier in this chapter we saw that the practical moral question for a "theocentric" construal of the world is, What is God enabling and requiring us to be and to do? Gustafson's answer, articulated in the first volume of *Ethics From a Theocentric Perspective*, is that we are to relate ourselves and all things in a manner appropriate to their relations to God. However, midway through the second volume of that work he amends both question and answer somewhat: "What is God enabling and requiring us, as *participants* in the patterns and processes of interdependence of life in the world, to be and to do? ... We, as participants, are to relate ourselves and all things in a manner appropriate to our and their relations to God" ([16], p. 146 – emphasis added).

This alteration is significant for what it emphasizes about Gustafson's anthropology and his view of human life in the world. From his perspective, human life is to be construed "in continuity with 'nature' as much as in distinction from it." We are radically *dependent* upon the rest of the natural world. But we are also radically *interdependent*; the relationship between human activity and the rest of the world is an "interactive" one ([14], pp. 282–83). In piety we can recognize our finitude, i.e., limits established by the divine governance for our agential capacities. We can also recognize the possibilities open to us – our individual and corporate capacities for action – within the divine ordering. Gustafson employs the model of human "participation" to emphasize that we are not simply "spectators" to life's patterns and processes of interdependence, but neither are we the "proprietor of creation" or "all-powerful emperor of the world." We are indeed *part* of a *whole* (or, actually various "wholes"). The traditional religious term most in accord with "participation," he writes, is "stewardship"; for that term also conveys the reality that we are "temporary, responsible custodians of, and contributors to, the realms in which we participate" ([16], p. 145).

Of course, we do not always construe ourselves and our world in this way. Gustafson observes that all humans experience the "human fault" in four aspects: misplaced confidence or trust ("idolatry"); misplaced valuations of objects of desire (wrongly ordered love); erroneous perceptions of things in their relations to each other ("corrupt" rationality); and the experience of unfulfilled duties and obligations (disobedience) ([14], p. 294). Following Augustine and Edwards, Gustafson describes these aspects of the human fault through the metaphor of "contraction" of the human spirit: contraction of our trust and loyalty; contraction of our loves and desires; contraction of our "vision"; and contraction of our moral interests ([14], pp. 304–306). The "correction" which is evoked and sustained in theocentric piety is, then, an "enlargement" of the soul and of our interests. Such a correction involves: (1) an alteration and enlargement of vision (such that we "see" more relevant "wholes" of life in which we function); (2) an alteration and enlargement of the "order of the heart" (in accordance with our experience of God's governing direction); and (3) different standards for determining proper human being and action, based upon the former corrections ([14], pp. 308–15).

Now, with respect to the last of these "corrections," Gustafson insists that theocentric piety is *not* manifest in a rule-centered legalism; indeed, the notion that human goodness rests in obedience to strict rules covering all cases can be a *restraint* upon true "consent" to the divine purposes. Theocentrism does not reject rules and principles altogether, but indicates a sense that they need to be general ones whose application "must be addressed to changing historical conditions." This is because it is not given to us to know inerrantly what the divine governance requires under some circumstances, and also because the divine governance is not an "immutable eternal order" but an *ordering*. Thus, rules and principles "have to be open to revision and extension in the light of alterations in natural, social, historical, cultural, and individual conditions" ([14], pp. 315–16).

A theocentric construal (and "correction" of affections and valuations) does not, then, issue in a rules-centered understanding of moral life. Nor can it assure the sense of moral certainty promised by many deontological (and utilitarian) moral theories:

It does not relieve the anxiety of taking risks; it does not eliminate the need sometimes to act unjustly for the sake of a wider justice; it does not resolve the deep ambiguities of moral choices in certain particular conditions; and it does not eliminate the possibility of genuine tragedy as a feature of human moral experience. It does not provide a bland assurance that something good will issue from every circumstance of what is injurious to human welfare, that every 'crucifixion' will issue in a glorious 'resurrection,' that all things work together for good for those who love God ([14], p. 316f.).

Indeed, one does not, from a theocentric perspective, develop an "ideal moral theory" at all. To do so, in Gustafson's view, would be to adopt the posture of ideal *spectator* – and one who claims to see and evaluate things from God's reference-point, to boot! ([16], p. 146). Instead, theocentric ethics is first and foremost a matter of *discernment*. For, discernment is the process through which we can reach some certitude (albeit not always certainty) about what God is enabling and requiring and about the appropriate relations to God of ourselves and all things ([14], p. 327).

Discernment is not simply perception; it is a qualitative, discriminating, interpretive process. Moral discernment begins with an "evaluative description" of the circumstances or occasion we face: "Either consciously or intuitively we depict that to which we feel affectively moved to respond." In so doing we make judgments about what information is salient to that particular situation, about what gives it explanatory coherence and what best indicates how and why it came to be. We also make judgements about what factors are morally relevant (i.e., about what is morally at stake) and about what features of the situation could be affected through powers available to us ([14], pp. 333–35).

Every evaluative description is made from a particular *perspective*, shaped by individual or communal inclination, training, and settled convictions. The range of factors taken to be important in a given situation is widened or narrowed by our perspective: e.g., the range of past causative or motivating factors and potential consequences in the future; the range of relationships among human and other beings involved; etc. ([14], pp. 335–36). (We have already noted, for instance, those limitations imposed upon evaluative descriptions by the "anthropocentric" perspective Gustafson criticizes so strongly.)

Interwoven with one's fundamental perspective are other factors which also affect moral discernment. Generalized beliefs about human nature and motivation, for instance, will color our evaluations of what responses (by others) are possible or probable. The moral principles and values to which we are committed will frame the range of responses we see as morally "fitting." And, of course, our attitudes and dispositions – our senses of duty, gratitude, hope, etc. – will color how we envision possibilities and obligations.[4]

Of course, these factors in the process of discernment are in large part matters of the events, environments, and webs of belief which "in-form" us (as Hauerwas has also argued, using somewhat different language). But Gustafson insists that they do not alone yield our particular discernments. For, moral discernment is fundamentally a reflective, rational activity: "It is reflection on one's own motives and desires." We reflectively sort through better or worse means and consequences of our responses. And we rationally choose the ends toward which we act; those ends "do not merely flow from the sorts of persons we are becoming."[5] Interestingly, though, Gustafson describes the final result of discernment as "an informed *intuition*":

[I]t is not the conclusion of a formally logical argument, a strict deduction from a single moral principle, or an absolutely certain result from the exercises of human 'reason' alone. There is a final moment of perception that sees the parts in relation to a whole, expresses sensibilities as well as reasoning, and is made in the conditions of human finitude ([14], p. 338; [6], p. 108).

Given this description of the process of moral discernment, then, what can be discerned through that process about the divine governance of all things? Gustafson replies, first, that the divine governance *cannot* be discerned in terms of a "timeless and changeless moral order." Discernment takes into account developments in culture, history, nature, society and self which imply that "ethics itself develops," that traditionally-held moral principles may need revision, extension of their application, or even radical alteration. Thus, theocentric ethics cannot have the normative certainty which some moral philosophers and Roman Catholic natural law theorists believe possible. Nor can the Bible reveal to us the moral details of the divine governance of *our* world, even though it is the record of a people of piety who discerned what was morally required of *them* under *their* particular natural and historical conditions ([14], p. 339).

Positively, what *can* be discerned about the divine governance are the necessary conditions – the "fundamental requisites" – for the development and sustenance of life (human personal, social, institutional and species life, and also the life of the natural world). These fundamental requisites form the "bases" for ethical reflection. And while they are necessarily discerned and expressed in very general and formal terms, they "establish the grounds of more particular and precise principles and general rules" and also "indicate the basic directions that more particular ordering and actions must take" ([14], pp. 339–40). Thus, while theocentric discernment rejects any static, immutable "order" of creation from which moral norms follow by simple rational deduction, our moral determinations of proper ends, right actions, and fitting aspirations nevertheless *are* grounded in "an objective 'reality' of which human life is a part" ([16], p. 8). In a formal sense, then, theocentric ethics shares some common ground with natural law theory – especially when contrasted with existentialist ethics or traditional divine-command theories of morality. Gustafson notes that the "major affinity" between his work and Thomas Aquinas's is the importance for theological ethics of an interpretation of the divine ordering of nature and of how finite and contingent things can "reveal" their relations to God ([16], pp. 44–45). (Of course, he also disagrees sharply with Aquinas's "anthropocentric" assumptions about human "essence" and with his *exitus et reditus* teleology of divine creation – [16], pp. 53–55.)

What Gustafson offers is, broadly speaking, a naturalistic (and experiential) theology and ethics which is not a traditional natural law theology but is nevertheless fundamentally teleological in character. Its *telos*, discovered in piety, is not eternal reunion or *beatitudo* with the Creator, but is rather the attainment of conformity (within our own conditions of finitude) with the divine purposes for all of creation. Basic inferences or indicators of what that conformity requires – i.e., the "fundamental requisites" for creation's well-being – are discovered through the process of discernment. Of course, discernment must also take us beyond the very general directionalities provided by the fundamental requisites (e.g., of *some* form of child rearing, of the basic requirements of ecosystems, etc.) to more specific values, ends, principles and sensibilities for guidance in particular decisions. This final step of discernment yields the "informed intuition" described above.

One helpful description of Gustafson's ethical method has been offered by John P. Reeder [29]. He refers to it as an ethic of "flourishing" (not only of humans but of all creation) that has three main dimensions. The first dimension is assent to God's purposes for the good of the whole creation. The second dimension is the notion of functional requisites, which theocentric discernment accepts as signs of God's ordering and governance of creation. In the "middle space" between these two dimensions, as it were, is the third dimension of "substantive notions which determine how the good of the whole and the good of parts within the whole are to be pursued, taking into account what we know about the prerequisites" ([29], pp. 128–29). Because the goods (the elements of "flourishing" of whole and of parts) to be ranked or weighted in this middle space are often incommensurate, and because we can discern no ultimate value or meta-principle for ranking them in all cases, theocentric decision-making is often tragic. Moral ambiguity cannot be avoided.

This is not to say, however, that theocentric ethics leads to "radical relativism." Gustafson insists that some "outer limits" or absolute prohibitions (e.g., of slavery or murder) are discernible. Moreover, relativism is limited by the "objective" factor of what we can know (albeit imperfectly) about the divine governance, and by "subjective" factors in accumulated human experience (e.g., knowledge of institutions necessary to meet basic conditions of human life, collective religious and ethical reflection about those conditions and about proper ends of human acts, cultural "ethos" and evaluations of history, literary disclosure of moral experience, etc.). Even so, these factors do not provide absolute moral certainty except in "relatively simple and extreme circumstances" ([14], pp. 340–41). All too often we cannot bring into harmony all of the ethically defensible values and claims we face; some of them must be sacrificed in favor of others.

Now, one other aspect of theocentric ethics meriting our attention at this point is Gustafson's treatment of "parts" and "wholes." For, he notes that what distinguishes his project from many others is its larger descriptive context (of persons, communities, species, events, and other things as parts of larger wholes). We must, he says, not only recognize the "wholes" in which we participate and which our choices will affect; we must also recognize and weigh the good of these wholes along with (and against) the individual goods of persons, groups, and things which are parts of them. An "interactional" model of human agency must reject both a strictly "organic" analogy of interrelationships (in which the organic whole is prior to, and deterministically produces, individuals) and a purely "contractual" model (in which individuals are primary, and freely choose and determine the nature and extent of larger wholes) ([14], pp. 292–93; [16], pp. 12–19). Theocentric ethics is not, then, a moral theory centered in natural (or derived) human rights and liberties. And Gustafson insists that, while his ethics gives great emphasis to the *consequences* of human action, it is not a utilitarian theory, either. For, in his view, utilitarianism emphasizes the good of "wholes" as *aggregations* of individual human goods: "it holds that any 'whole' that has to be taken into account exists for the ends of its individual members" ([16], p. 109).

Theocentric ethics, on the other hand, sees the goods of relevant wholes (e.g., the family) as goods in and of themselves, and not merely the sum of the goods of their individual members. As Gustafson puts it at one point, the common good and the good of its individuals are "reciprocal, but not harmonious." One result of this, he suggests, is that his proposal, while recognizing the moral importance of individual consents, could nevertheless warrant "paternalism" (or restraint of participation in some defined whole) more readily in some circumstances than would the classic utilitarian view, and certainly more readily than contractarian theories ([16], p. 110).

Of course, any discussion of "wholes" raises conceptual questions with respect to the *scope* of wholes to be taken into account, and for whose sake they should be considered. Gustafson's answers to these two questions, he tells us, distinguish his work from that of "most other Western moral theorists." As for the scope of wholes, he admits that no person can perceive, conceive or respond to "*the* whole." But the various sciences can help us to know about and interpret natural patterns of interdependence and causal relationships which enlarge the temporal and spatial wholes we can describe and consider. And a theocentric commitment to the well-being of the whole creation, even in the abstract, presses us to expand the scope of wholes we take into account in our normative ethics. The family and the community are obvious examples, but so are our national and international economies, human and other species, the ecosphere, etc. In short, theocentric ethics requires that we extend our perception of, and commitment to, a broader range of wholes than merely the collectives of human interests which have dominated Western ethical theories.

Similarly, it is clear from what we have seen thus far that we cannot conceive of the whole as being "*only* or even *ultimately* for the sake of our part." A theocentric construal does not allow us to see our good – individual, community, or species – as the good ultimately served by the whole creation. Of course, we cannot fully define what "*the* good of *the* whole" really is (except, in religious terms, that its purpose is to glorify God). In our finitude, we have to think in terms of the goods of particular wholes, recognizing that those goods are often incommensurable and that our choices will be tragic ones. The notion of "the common good" is a useful conceptual tool, in Gustafson's view, but theocentric ethics must avoid the extremes of either its "organic" or its individualistic versions. We will not find any easy resolution between the claims of totalities and individual claims of fairness and self-determination. Finally, however, our central focus in moral decision-making must be upon what we can discern of the good of the wholes at stake ([16], pp. 17–19).

In summary, then, Gustafson avers that his theocentric construal of the world

... requires that parts be interpreted in relation to relevant wholes, and that the common good of various wholes is the object of proper concern not only for the sake of the parts but also for the sake of those wholes. It follows from this that theocentric ethics will be weighted more readily, in circumstances of conflict between the claims of parts and the whole, on claims for the common good of a whole ([16], p. 19).

Now, reflecting upon Gustafson's proposal as it has been described here, we can see that it is a complex blend of several interrelated themes. Central to the project, of course, is the theme of religious affectivity – particularly *piety*. Our ability to discern "the way things really and ultimately are" in the divine ordering depends upon our affective powers as well as our rational powers. Practically, theocentric ethics requires more than a natural law commitment to a particular hierarchy of values, more than a set of specific rules of practice derived from *agape* or "covenant-faithfulness," and more than an identification of our stories with those of Jesus and the Church. It requires an understanding of ourselves as interactive participants in the divine ordering of the whole creation, which exists, in turn, for God's purposes and God's glorification. Thus, it requires that we avail ourselves not only of orthodox doctrines and principles but also of evidences and inferences from other sources (e.g., the sciences) in discerning normative patterns of divine governance. Finally, theocentric ethics demands that, in relating ourselves and all things in a manner appropriate to their relations to God, we must broaden our moral vision and perspective in order to recognize and pursue the good of relevant "wholes" as well as those of individual (or aggregate) persons and things.

The tasks of being and doing, then, are neither simple nor objectively certain from a theocentric perspective; those tasks require the "senses" and consideration of manifold dimensions of human experience. So, one should not expect from Gustafson many simplistic answers to "What would you do if . . ." sorts of questions. Even so, the remaining sections of this chapter will attempt to cast further light on Gustafson's project by examining some of his responses to our representative issues in medical ethics: refusal of life-prolonging treatment by competent patients; treatment choices for severely handicapped newborns; and the use of children in nontherapeutic medical research.

3. DISCERNMENT AND THE REFUSAL OF LIFE-PROLONGING TREATMENT

Compared with McCormick, Ramsey and Hauerwas, Gustafson has written relatively little on the specific topic of competent persons' refusals of life-prolonging treatment. It is not surprising, of course, that he has avoided recommending any blanket moral judgement or policy on the subject, given his description of the range of cognitive and affective factors to be considered in discerning a fitting response within one's particular circumstances.

So we must proceed in this section (and the two remaining sections of this chapter) by examining his occasional comments on the issue(s) and, more fundamentally, his analysis of "points to be considered" (a phrase he borrows from Karl Barth) in moral discernments of this sort.

In keeping with the format of previous chapters, let us begin with some of Gustafson's views on the theological significance of human life and death. Many of his explorations of life-and-death issues are prefaced with a brief quotation from Barth: "Life is no second God, and therefore the respect due it cannot rival the reverence owed to God" (see, e.g., [8], p. 60; [21]). Human physical life is not, in Gustafson's view, of absolute value. Nevertheless, it is something to be valued for its own sake, since it is the "indispensable condition for human values and valuing" ([4], p. 140). The moral burden of proof, then, rests with those who would take or deny life. But that is not an insurmountable burden.

A religious qualification of our understanding of human life's value suggests several important points of reference. First, because we are indeed dependent upon the author and source of all life, we should accept created life as a *gift* and respond in gratitude. (As we will see, however, Gustafson does not believe that gratitude can or should *always* be our *dominant* sense of, or response to, our own created existence.) Second, our valuation of life must recognize the finitude and deformity of our existence; only God is absolute, and we must not absolutize that which is relative. Third, we are accountable to God for the ways in which we care for, preserve, sustain and cultivate life. And, fourth, as we participate in the created order, we must be "responsive to the developments and purposes which are being made possible for [us] under the power and gifts of life from God" ([4], pp. 142–43).

One clear inference from these points is that we must have genuine respect for what God has created and for those avenues of life-preservation open to us through the divine governance. Theocentric ethics does not, then, give rise to any obstructionist or anti-progressive attitude toward research and development of life-prolonging technologies. At the same time, however, medical scientists should be reminded that "death is as integral an aspect of human life as it is of all other biologic species'." Thus, technological developments primarily aimed at prolonging life "should be seriously questioned if the ultimate result is destined to be a grotesque, fragmented, or inordinately expensive existence" [21]. Gustafson is never quite as specific as, say, Ramsey or McCormick in defining what sort of existence would be "grotesque, fragmented, or inordinately expensive." But he insists that death is *not* the "enemy" of the sick or of health professionals; rather, their proper enemies are fear, anxiety, disability, disease and discomfort. Indeed, sensitive, perceptive physicians will try to guide their patients (the relatively well along with the severely ill and handicapped) to "a perspective in which the preservation of life is not their God" [21].

Now, we should recall here that Gustafson finds no scientific or experiential evidence for Christian beliefs in resurrection destiny or 'life after death.' So, he is not claiming that death should be chosen as "friend" or as a positive, affirming alternative to the value of life. He is claiming instead that physical life may be perceived correctly as losing its human value when other human values (for which life is the indispensable condition) are unrealizable within it. Put differently, this means that our sense of gratitude for the gift of life need not always be expressed morally in a willingness to continue in it. Ramsey and Hauerwas, both of whom draw inferences from the metaphor of life-as-gift, would agree that our gratitude does not require artificial prolongation of life in the face of suffering when death is inevitable and relatively imminent. But such choices, they tell us, are really choices about how to *live* in one's final days; they are not direct choices *for death*. The latter choices, on the other hand, amount to ingratitude ("throwing the gift back in the face of the giver") or failure of trust. This sort of moral distinction on their part is the locus of a significant contrast between their moral judgements and Gustafson's. For, in Gustafson's theocentric perspective, some deliberate decisions for death ('suicide,' whether by commission or omission) are not only understandable and excusable but also *justifiable*.

Suicide is one of the four topical issues Gustafson explores in the second volume of *Ethics from a Theocentric Perspective* as illustrations of theocentric discernment. After surveying several "benchmark" arguments (from Barth, Aquinas, Kant, Mill and Sidgewick) about the morality of suicide, Gustafson goes on to examine "conditions of the human spirit" which can make suicide appear as an attractive choice. Specifically, he focuses on several forms of "the sense of tribulation, affliction, or despair": a sense of impossibility, or "fatedness"; a deep conflict of loyalties; a sense of aimlessness or purposelessness; isolation from necessary patterns of mutual interdependence; and an excessive sense of moral scrupulosity ([16], pp. 201–206). From a theocentric perspective, he concludes, our first responsibility is to make suicide an unnecessary or less apparent option for those facing such affliction by attending to the patterns and processes of our interdependence, thus sustaining others and the relationships which make life worthwhile for all of us.

A second responsibility is to "restrain persons from the act [of suicide] if we have opportunity to do so." Now, this responsibility, cited several times by Gustafson, would seem to amount to a requirement that suicide attempts be interdicted whenever and wherever possible. But that is not the case, for he goes on to describe yet a third responsibility which follows from theocentric discernment:

Alas, for all too many persons there are good and realistic grounds for the deepest despair: persons facing unrelievable pain and suffering of body and spirit, persons facing the bleakness of continuous poverty and unemployment, persons facing the loss of simple human dignity. No ringing ideals, no cogent argument for an imperative of a duty to oneself, no charge of self-justification, and no counsel of possibilities will bring relief or hope. To deaths of such persons by suicide one must consent. The powers that bear down upon them are greater than the powers that sustain them. Neither moralists nor God ought to be their judge ([16], p. 209).

In other words, there are morally justifiable suicides – cases in which interference (or even negative judgement) would not be fitting. And that category would include many justifiable choices for suicide by means of omissions (refusals of treatment). But what about the difficult task of discerning *which* choices for death fall outside our responsibility to intervene and which do not? Gustafson does not go so far as to offer clear and concrete criteria for distinguishing among them. Moral discernment is, after all, very much context-related. However, his concrete examples do offer some hints about the directions of his own (albeit general) discernments. Against Kant's argument that taking one's life to avoid misery is not justifiable, he responds that persons facing "what is reasonably perceived to be unbearable and unrelievable suffering" are in no way accountable for those sufferings, and their decisions to seek the relief of death "for their own sake and for that of others" can be not only understandable and excusable but also justifiable choices. Yet he goes on to say that the full nature and context of the suffering must be taken into account. So, for instance, the case of an adolescent boy "whose aim in life is to be a great athlete and who is permanently disabled by an accident" is "quite different" from that of a person who has undergone "years of suffering, whose capacities to value life and contribute to others have been largely spent, and for whom there are no courses of action available which can relieve the suffering." Likewise, the treatment-refusal cases of an aged person who is ill or the patient on renal dialysis who can no longer tolerate its effects are different from that of a young adult "whose injury precludes that one aspiration can be fulfilled but does not rule out others." In the latter case, from Gustafson's perspective, medical intervention (even against the patient's will) would be morally warranted because of the patient's present and future "possibilities for participation in life for his own sake and for the roles he can have in human communities." (Here Gustafson cites his agreement with Thomas Aquinas that when a member of a human community "who has prospects of functioning in significant ways in life" is lost to the community, this deprivation "violates a common good" and thus is a warrant for intervention.) ([16], pp. 214–15).

Now, several facets of Gustafson's analysis are clearly reflected in these exemplary comments and comparisons. First, as noted earlier, he insists that a patient's rejection of life-prolonging treatment based upon a desire and intent to die (i.e., suicide) is not necessarily any less justifiable than a rejection based upon the burdensomeness of treatment in one's remaining life. A deliberate choice for death, for one's own sake or for the sake of others, can indeed be morally proper.

Second, however, a patient's autonomous treatment-refusal, whether based upon a desire for death or upon the treatment's burdensomeness, is at best only presumptively binding upon others. Care-givers' choices for medical intervention are not morally circumscribed by the patient's autonomous acceptance of them. From a theocentric perspective it is certainly correct to respect persons' capacities for agency; but "persons are more than their capacities for agency." We are to respect persons "not merely as individuals but as 'members one of another' in their communities . . . Indeed, when one sees how restricted is the range in which autonomy is exercised, and when one sees how the exercise of agency is dependent upon and limited by biological, social, cultural, and other conditions, respect *only* for autonomy can be viewed as denigrating" ([14], p. 291 – emphasis added).

Third, moral warrants for non-consensual, life-prolonging interventions may be based on paternalistic evaluations of the patient's own good – i.e., a positive medical prognosis that includes the patient's "present and future possibilities for participation in life for his own sake." However, they may also be drawn from notions of "common good," from a consideration of "the roles [the patient] can have in human communities." In other words, forced intervention may be justifiable if the patient's (immediate) death would diminish the community's well-being or deprive it of significant functional participation. Gustafson is aware, of course, that such a suggestion may sound rather utilitarian to some. But he insists (as we saw in the previous section of this chapter) that a genuinely theocentric perspective cannot limit its focus to an individualistic construal of what is in fact our "interactional" life in the world. It must also recognize and weigh the good of relevant "wholes" – a good which may not coincide with self-perceived individual goods, or even the aggregate of those individual goods.

Now, in many respects Gustafson's views on autonomous treatment-refusals parallel those of McCormick, Ramsey and Hauerwas. All affirm the general premise that human life is a divine gift and, all other things being equal, a value to be perserved. But all agree that some choices against prolonging life medically are morally appropriate choices. All affirm a basic moral obligation to respect the agency and self-determination of persons, including the sick and dying. And yet all four offer moral justification for overriding autonomous treatment-refusals in some circumstances.

Despite these convergences among the four positions, however, we have seen that Gustafson's differs from the other three in at least two significant respects. The first has to do with his concern for the good of "wholes": he is the only one of the four to suggest that the community's good *per se* can furnish a sufficient moral warrant for enforced life-prolonging treatment. Hauerwas may be moving in the same general direction when he describes the positive obligations the dying have toward their supporting communities; nevertheless, explicit assertions that the community's flourishing would justify enforced medical prolongation of life are conspicuously absent from his writings (and those of Ramsey and McCormick).

Second, Gustafson's theology leads him to conclusions about the moral legitimacy of some choices for suicide that are not echoed in previous chapters of this study. Despite his agreement that human life is a gift to be received with gratitude, Gustafson is alone in his further assertion that the powers bestowing the gift may also render it unbearable, in which case there is legitimate reason to "quarrel with God" or even to hold "enmity" toward God. Indeed, he may have been accusing Ramsey, McCormick and Hauerwas (and many other Christian thinkers) of theological short-sightedness when he wrote:

That God not only does not guarantee the good of the afflicted persons, but also that conditions of possibility to meet their reasonable interests do not exist should raise again traditional theological difficulties that are sometimes easily ignored. The experiences of persons from which reasonably follows their self-destruction . . . are crucibles in which claims about the benevolence and beneficence of God are severely tested. Finally one has to consent to the reality that the powers that bring life into being do not always sustain it but can lead to its untimely and tragic destruction ([16], p. 216).

In summary, then, Gustafson's account of theocentric discernment about treatment refusals would appear to be less rule-limited – and more broad-ranging in its interpretation of relevant "wholes" to be considered and of the Christian metaphor of life-as-gift – than the other accounts described in this study. As we have seen, one practical result is that his approach yields a comparatively wider range of considerations that may favor restricting others' autonomous choices for death, but also a wider range of considerations favoring non-judgemental acquiescence in such choices. Yet the tension inherent in this result is virtually inescapable (and quite typical of Gustafson's topical analyses), given the range of "points to consider" (from both cognitive and affective sources) upon which theocentric discernment depends.

4. DISCERNMENT AND TREATMENT DECISIONS FOR DEFECTIVE NEONATES

Prior to the Bloomington "Baby Doe" case of 1982, perhaps the most widely-discussed instance of selective non-treatment of a 'defective' baby had been the nearly identical Johns Hopkins case (cited in Chapter 1). In that instance, the parents of a newborn with duodenal atresia had refused the relatively simple corrective surgery for that problem, apparently because the child had also been diagnosed with Down's syndrome (or, in the popular language of the time, 'mongolism'). Because the baby could not be fed with his intestine blocked, he died of starvation/dehydration at 15 days of age.

One of the earliest commentaries on the Johns Hopkins case (and surely the most widely reprinted) was Gustafson's 1973 essay, "Mongolism, Parental

Desires, and the Right to Life" [5]. That work remains his only extensive discussion of neonatal treatment decisions; thus it provides perhaps the best starting point for our consideration here. Unlike many other discussions of neonatal treatment choices, Gustafson's analysis of the Johns Hopkins case does not seek to establish and defend a set of criteria for morally appropriate choices and then apply them to the case at hand. Instead, he attempts to interpret what is at stake in the case from within the various *perspectives* involved – those of the mother and father, the physicians and the nurses. In focusing on agential perspectives in this way, he seeks an understanding of their discernments, of how they may have come to weight relatively their own valuations of a Down's-afflicted life, parental 'rights' to choose what they desire for their children, the infant's own 'right to life,' legal ramifications of choices made, and other circumstances which present (and limit) the genuine possibilities for action.

For example, Gustafson explores the mother's "negative feeling" about retardation and its sources in our intelligence-valuing society; her concern that she would be incapable of giving the infant the care and affection he would require; her assumption (based in part on her professional experiences as a nurse) of a "factual distinction" between a "normal" infant and a "mongoloid" sufficient morally to ground differential access to the same life-prolonging surgery; and her assumption that it would be "unfair" to her two other children to raise them with a Down's child. These factors so "qualify" her perception of herself, her circumstances, and her possibilities vis-à-vis the infant that they outweigh, for her, any sense that her child's very existence might lay upon her an "unconditional moral claim" to the necessary conditions for sustenance ([5], pp. 533–38).

After examining in like manner probable factors in other involved agents' perspectives, Gustafson then proposes "a different moral point of view" from which to make an evaluative judgement. This alternative perspective would, he writes, "recast" the moral dilemma by giving a different weight to two crucial factors: the desires of the parents would be seen as less morally determinative in and of themselves; and the claims of the mongoloid infant to life would be given greater weight. The parents and physicians would recognize that there are "things one ought to do even when one has no immediate feelings about doing them, no immediate strong desire to do them." They would also see that "mongolism is not sufficiently deviant from what is normatively human to merit death" ([5], p. 549). Thus, they would no doubt conclude that the corrective surgery should be performed.

In defending this re-weighting of parental desires and infant claims to life, Gustafson's initial epistemological appeal is to "common experience" – particularly the experience of family relationships – and the natural piety evoked therein. Family is the earliest "school" for the senses of dependence, gratitude, obligation, remorse and repentance, direction, and possibility – all of which ground piety and, thus, theology and ethics ([16], p. 173). Our children, because of their very existence as individually valuable humans and because of their relationship of dependence upon us, evoke in their parents a sense of obligation not contingent upon immediate parental desires:

> I would argue that the fact that we brought our children into being lays a moral obligation on my wife and me to sustain and care for them to the best of our ability. They did not choose to be; and their being is dependent, both causally and in other ways, upon us. In the relationship of dependence, there is a claim of them over against us . . . Their claims are independent of our desires to fulfill them.[6]

Of course, their claims are also manifold; and conditions of possibility may not be present for meeting all of those claims. But certainly the most basic sort of filial dependence – and parental obligation – involves the sustenance necessary for life itself. And that obligation is not conditioned by their IQ scores, their physical attributes, or by any predictions about whether they will become the persons we want them to become ([5], p. 551). The presumption, then, "is always in favor of sustaining life through ordinary means."[7] This may indeed prove costly and/or burdensome for parents and other family members. But the sense of obligation evoked in family life teaches us that "self-denial is not a supererogatory norm; it is a moral necessity for common life" ([16], p. 171).

Further, the sense of obligation evoked by the infant's dependence is not limited to the family context: "The dependence relationship holds for the physicians as well as the parents in this case." Human life presents a claim for preservation that grounds a presumptive moral obligation for those with the capacity and ability to save it ([5], p. 552). That obligation is not contingent, then, upon the physician's own desires concerning handicapped infants or upon his/her wish to respect the parents' express desires.

On the other hand, though, within the perspective Gustafson describes one would not view the obligation to sustain infant life as unexceptionable. There are circumstances, he writes, in which we "cannot avoid using qualities and potential consequences in the determination of what might be justifiable exceptions to the presumption of the right to life on the part of any infant – indeed, any person." As we might expect, he does not specify particular divergences from "normal" (or potential consequences for the infant's continued existence) sufficient to justify decisions not to treat. Instead he simply asserts that parents and physicians are not obliged to sustain the life of an infant judged to be a "monstrosity" ([5], pp. 553–54). However, some general clues about his own recommended "points to consider" emerge from his explanation of why he would "draw the line on a different side of mongolism" than the physicians did in the Johns Hopkins case.

First of all, to withhold life-sustaining treatment on the basis of intelligence alone is a "simplistic" over-valuation of only one aspect of our existence.

To view intelligence as determinative over all other qualities is to "impoverish the richness and variety of human life." After all, the mongoloid infant still has potentialities for "satisfaction in life, for fulfilling his limited capacities, for happiness [and] for providing the occasions of meaningful . . . experience for others" ([5], p. 555).

Further, Gustafson would assess the significance of suffering in a different manner than was apparent among the actors in the Johns Hopkins case. We must ask ourselves, he writes, at what cost to others can we justify avoiding suffering for ourselves? Is the avoidance of potential economic and emotional suffering of family and care-givers sufficient to justify the cost of an infant's life? And, finally, does the prospective suffering appear to be *bearable* for those who will suffer? Gustafson appeals here to the religious qualification of his own convictions, to the belief that to be human "is to have a vocation, a calling, and the calling of each of us is 'to be for others' at least as much as 'to be for ourselves'" ([5], pp. 555–56).

One might infer from these suggestions that the prospect of *unbearable* suffering (which is, of course, not only a matter of prediction but also of *attitude*) of those involved could be seen as a legitimate factor in neonatal treatment decisions. But the 'burden of proof' would certainly rest with the one who would try to justify its primacy over the basic (albeit non-absolute) value of the infant's continued life.

As for his other locus of concerns – the infant's potentialities for satisfaction, fulfillment, or happiness in life – Gustafson may be suggesting something like McCormick's criterion of "relational potential" (see Chapter 2) as a basis for discernments about the value of continued life to the infant himself. It would seem, at least, that an infant with severe cognitive, motor and sensory deficiencies, who faces at best a short and painful life, would not have the "potentialities" Gustafson cites as warrants for preserving the life of the Johns Hopkins baby. Even so, however, we should note that he would reject McCormick's derivation of that criterion from any neat, objective hierarchy of goods (*ordo bonorum*). Such clear deductions are, he insists, simply unavailable to us. When we step onto the "sponge" of considering life's "qualities" we need to face "their variety, their complexity, the abrasiveness of one against the other" ([5], p. 555).

Finally, too, our discernments in this matter must encompass more than simply the question of whether a severely defective child should be allowed to die. In circumstances where that question is judged in the affirmative, then we must also discern our responsibility in *how* that death comes about. Gustafson (like Hauerwas) is critical of the often-defended moral distinction between allowing an infant's death and causing it. If a conscientious decision has been reached in favor of not prolonging the infant's life, he asks, then for whose advantage do we justify allowing a lingering (and perhaps painful) death but refuse to justify hastening that death? In his estimation, it is to the advantage of those agents making the choice, not to the infant's advantage. The "rigorist" who employs such a distinction to hide from the practical consequences of his/her choice "avoids a kind of moral culpability at the cost of the suffering of another." From a theocentric perspective, however,

> ... the dependence of the infant on the care of others implies that *if* the intention to have it die is morally justifiable, then, for the sake not of the agent but of the recipient, it would be morally permissible to intervene actively to hasten its death ([16], p. 314).

Interestingly, Gustafson admits that this claim is subject to a "counter-argument" from within his perspective as well. For, theocentric discernment must also include consideration of relevant larger wholes, including the community and its flourishing. So, in the issue at hand, discernment must take into account the possible long-range adverse consequences of any death-hastening acts for the "general respect for life" in our society and for other patients' attitudes of confidence in their physicians. After all, neonatal treatment decisions – like all other moral discernments – cannot be isolated from the larger contexts of our lives together in communities.

As we might expect by now, Gustafson offers no neat resolution of the tension between these considerations. Instead, he simply concludes that any "rigoristic adherence" to the allowing-to-die vs. killing distinction will have morally "mixed" consequences, that we should and must face ambiguity in making these choices, and that involved agents "should be required to give their reasons" for whatever choice is made ([16], p. 315).

Of course, Gustafson notes, many choices concerning life-prolonging treatment for a defective infant are irreducibly tragic – all available options may appear cruel or irresponsible. And whatever general rules or criteria may emerge from our perspectives cannot alone lead us to a 'fitting' discernment in every case. We must also be open, in an attitude of piety, to those senses of gratitude, obligation, remorse and repentance, etc., that qualify what we see, the possibilities and "boundary conditions" of our choices, and the relevant "wholes" for which we are responsible within the divine ordering of creation.

5. NONTHERAPEUTIC PEDIATRIC RESEARCH: THE GOOD OF PARTS AND OF WHOLES

Children's involvement in nontherapeutic medical research is a topic upon which Gustafson has not offered substantial commentary. Most of his references to it appear in methodological discussions or as illustrative examples cited within analyses of broader issues. Nevertheless, his "points to consider" on the matter do offer, either explicitly or by inference, clear indications about his perspective. Indeed, his discussions reveal specific and marked contrasts between his discernment and those of Ramsey and McCormick.

To begin with, he finds Ramsey's "love monism" (Gustafson's term) an insufficient basis for genuinely theocentric discernment. Recall that Ramsey's approach begins by drawing together biblical themes of "covenant-fidelity" and *agape*; the resultant central norm of covenant-love then becomes the source from which all moral principles and rules derive their meaning. And among the derivative rules especially pertinent to medical research are "do not harm" and "always obtain the informed consent of the research subject" (the "cardinal canon of loyalty" between researcher and subject). Since children presumably are unable to give a fully competent, voluntary, informed consent, Ramsey concludes that "in-principled love" would exclude them from nontherapeutic medical research altogether (though not from all therapeutic research).

Now, Gustafson is critical of this analysis on several counts. First, and most obviously, his theocentric approach cannot be confined and limited by Ramsey's biblically-derived love-monism. For, in piety we sense, and develop attitudes toward, the powers that bear down upon us and sustain us in many different ways, not all of which are reducible to Ramsey's understanding of covenant-love. Granted, Ramsey himself avers that we discern covenant fidelity's importance not only from Scripture but also from our *experience* of covenants in our daily lives; and Gustafson might well agree with this in large measure. Even so, he would no doubt counter that neither our particular experiences of covenant nor the biblical witness to God's covenantal activities (toward *that* people at *that* time) are sufficient to evoke the range of sensibilities grounding our responses to what God is enabling and requiring us to be and do as participants now, in the *whole* of creation.

Second, Gustafson finds inadequate the rule-centered "legalism" of Ramsey's ethical method. Adherence to strict, unexceptionable rules of practice can be a restraint to theocentric piety's true "consent" to the divine purposes. The divine goverance of creation is not fully knowable by us, and is not an immutable and eternal "order," anyway, but rather a dynamic "ordering." This does not mean that nothing is prohibited; rather, it suggests that our discriminating judgements may be "directed but not fully determined" by general rules ([16], p. 315).

Not surprisingly, then, Gustafson takes issue with Ramsey's rule-based rejection of any and all nontherapeutic pediatric research. There are, he insists, occasions in which the prospective benefits to others may warrant medical experimentation with young subjects for whom no individual medical benefit is foreseen. The "crucial theological difference" between his perspective and Ramsey's, Gustafson observes, is in "the emphasis that I give to God as the power that creates new possibilities for well-being in events of nature and history, including the possibilities that emerge in . . . the development of biological knowledge" ([8], p. 44).

This emphasis does not deny the moral significance of personal autonomy and the (presumptive) rule of informed consent. Indeed, Gustafson considers honoring persons' capacities for self-determination to be very much a part of relating to them "in a manner appropriate to their relations to God" ([16], p. 308). At the same time, however, he insists that ethical analyses of biomedical research focusing almost exclusively on informed consent are "ethically shortsighted"; they reflect the narrow anthropocentrism and individualism of much of our culture ([16], pp. 276, 310). From a theocentric perspective we can recognize that there may be occasions in which experimentation's prospective health-preserving benefits for large numbers of others and for future generations cannot be fulfilled within a stringent adherence to the principle of individual autonomy. Thus, arguments can be made for "overriding the protection of individual liberty for the sake of benefits to others or to a justifiable common good if all possible alternatives have been exhausted."[8]

Of course, the rule of informed consent is not the only norm invoked in the pediatric research debate, anyway. On Gustafson's reading, Ramsey's primary research concern has to do not so much with informed consent as with another love-derived maxim, "do not harm" – which, in his formulation, almost becomes "take no risks" ([16], p. 89; see also [8], pp. 44–47). And the only risks with which Ramsey concerns himself are those prospective research risks to be borne by healthy child-subjects. From Gustafson's viewpoint, however, we must broaden our perspective to take into account other attendant risks as well, such as the risk of depriving other persons (and future generations) of beneficial therapy by restricting research too severely ([16], p. 89). Or, put differently, we have no guarantee that restraints upon research by the maxim "do not harm" (to particular individuals or species) will actually fulfill "the well-being of creation" ([8], p. 47). And from a theocentric perspective we must consider possibilities – even risk-imposing possibilities – for fulfilling the well-being of larger wholes, for serving the common good. That sort of consideration is, he notes, already a part of our understanding of societal responsibility in some areas. By way of example, he draws an analogy between (potential) research risks and those risks we already impose through military conscription:

In wartime presumably the enemy is an "unjust aggressor" against one's own nation; by weak analogy a preventable disease is an aggressor against the health of the community. It is arguable, at least, that where the risk of death is not as high as it is during combat, or where the maximum harm falls short of the risk of death, there are grounds for putting some [non-consenting] persons at risk for the sake of prospective benefits to others ([16], p. 309; see also [8], pp. 45–46).

This passage makes clear once again Gustafson's conviction, contra Ramsey, that neither the rule of informed consent nor a rule against imposing (non-consensual) risks can be elevated to the status of *sine qua non* in medical research – even in pediatric research. (Implicit in it, too, is a rejection of Ramsey's underlying interpretation of all nontherapeutic research participation as a matter of purely voluntary, supererogatory "charity.") Rather, from a theocentric perspective the well-being of relevant "wholes" may warrant the imposition of some risk upon interdependent individuals who are parts of those wholes – even if they cannot (or will not) consent to those risks.

Now, Gustafson's use of the analogy between research participation and military conscription offers an interesting point of contact between his discussion of pediatric research and McCormick's. For, both of them use this analogy to show how our society already accepts the moral judgement that some risks may be imposed upon individuals, even upon non-volunteers, for the sake of the community's common good. (Further, both define "common good" as a collective value which is not an aggregate of individual goods but rather the good of the community as an entity; the community's well-being or flourishing does not rest, then, simply on a calculation of the greatest satisfaction for the greatest number of citizens.) As for their conclusions, both affirm what Ramsey denies: that nontherapeutic research involving children is morally justifiable under some circumstances.

Despite these similarities, however, there are crucial differences between Gustafson's and McCormick's perspectives on the matter (and between their substantive conclusions). McCormick begins with the natural law premise that individuals ought to choose in favor of those goods definitive of their own growth and flourishing; and the good of natural sociality entails seeking others' flourishing, too, at least where that is possible without causing any great risk to oneself. In the case of minimal-risk, high prospect-of-benefit nontherapeutic research, this 'ought' translates into a natural duty of social justice, of bearing one's own minimal share of the research burden so that all may flourish. So, he argues, a child *would consent* to participate in low-risk/high-benefit nontherapeutic research, if he were able, because he reasonably *ought* to do so.

Gustafson, on the other hand, would question whether we can derive such a clear and specific duty from the good of natural sociality – or whether we can even perceive that good as McCormick defines it. He comes close to McCormick's language of natural duties when he writes that there is "an ordering activity in life, with its impositions of duties and obligations, its assignment of tasks and the requirement of their fulfillment, which is part of God's purpose for men" ([4], p. 148). And he would no doubt applaud McCormick's insistence upon 'updating' traditional Aristotelian-Thomistic understandings of essential human 'ends' (and our 'means' of attaining them) through our increased knowledge of physical and social sciences. Nevertheless, Gustafson's notion of the divine "ordering" of creation is quite different from McCormick's *ordo bonorum*. He does not perceive anything like natural law theory's clear hierarchy of values, essences, and human *teloi*, culminating in eternal *beatitudo* for the individual; indeed, the single, unambiguous *telos* he cites for all creation is the *glorification of God*. Thus, his normative assertion that we are to "relate ourselves and all things in a manner appropriate to our and their relations to God" is not equivalent to McCormick's assertion that we should always seek to attain the highest available good in the hierarchy of values.

In this sense, then, Gustafson cannot begin with McCormick's assumption that the highest objective value available in any situation is also good-for-me. He would no doubt be uncomfortable with McCormick's derivation of a child's presumed consent to research participation from his/her *own* good of natural sociality, premised upon some essential connection between the common good and the individual's good. For, from a theocentric perspective we see in our own interdependence that the relations between parts and wholes are "not necessarily harmonious," that the common good of a whole "is never in perfect harmony with justifiable goods of its parts" ([16], p. 302). Tragically, we must often choose between the conflicting goods of parts and of wholes without the moral comfort of believing our choices to be in the service of both – except, of course, insofar as we see those choices to be in the service of the divine ordering, the *telos* of all creation.

This difference in perspective yields a marked difference in substantive conclusions, too. Because of McCormick's particular correlation of personal flourishing with that of others (in the natural good of sociality), his derived duty of research participation is necessarily quite limited. It cannot require (or presume) of anyone a willingness to accept more than "minimal" research risks for the sake of others' flourishing. Any acceptance of risks beyond that is a matter of the personal good of "expressed charity," of possible denial of one's own physical flourishing for the sake of another, which cannot be generalized as a natural moral *obligation*. Thus, we can reasonably presume that children would consent to nontherapeutic experimentation *only* if the subject-risk is quite minimal (and the prospective knowledge-benefits substantial.)

In Gustafson's approach, however, we cannot begin by deriving the child-subject's own research obligation and then go on to explain how and when we can allow (or help) the child to meet that obligation. In fact, he rarely mentions the obligations of individual research subjects at all (except to observe, in a general sense, that all of us have duties or obligations to advance the well-being of relevant wholes). Instead, he consistently approaches the issue of research participation from the stance of the community – e.g., by asking when we can justify *imposing* research risks upon individual research subjects for the sake of the common good. The moral dilemma of using children in nontherapeutic research is not resolved, then, simply by a rational presumption of what the child-subject would or would not consent to. Rather, we must choose among the genuinely conflicting goods – individual and communal – at stake. And without any neat derivation of specific individual obligations concerning research participation, we are also left without the clear moral *limits* of those obligations vis-à-vis the needs and expectations of others.[9]

Not surprisingly, then, the most significant difference between Gustafson's and McCormick's conclusions has to do with the justification of risks for healthy subjects of nontherapeutic research. While McCormick insists upon "minimal risk" or "no significant risk" as the outer limit for any non-consenting subject, we have seen that Gustafson might be willing to justify risks approaching those of military combat, at least where the maximal potential harm is less than death and the prospective benefit to others is great. His rationale for such a limit is not entirely clear. What is clear, though, is his insistence that neither the self-determination nor the protection-from-risk of the potential research subject is an absolute value; that the common good, including progress in clinical medicine, becomes a very weighty value when seen in terms of the wellbeing of the *creation*; that discernments of this sort are fraught with ambiguity and are not subject to simple, formulaic solutions; and that our choices will often be tragic ones.

In summary, Gustafson's discernments in the area of pediatric experimentation appear more ready to impose subject-risks for the sake of medical progress than do any of the others examined in previous chapters. The primary reason for this lies in his understanding of what we are responsible to and for: as "participants in the patterns and processes of interdependence of life in the world" our responsibility is to relate ourselves and all things "in a manner appropriate to their relations to God" ([16], p. 146). Our senses of the powers that bear down upon and sustain us as participants include the sense of *possibility* as well as senses of gratitude, dependence, etc. Thus, a part of our responsibility – a part of "relating" ourselves and all things in creation appropriately – lies in transforming our sense of the possible into (literally) the art of the possible. Certainly the protection of individuals from experimental risks or threats to their autonomy is a part of the relating required of us, but so is the protection of communities and future generations from the risks of diseases whose treatment/cure stand before us as research possibilities. These values can and do come into conflict. And while the rules we develop for adjudicating among them can be useful guideposts for our discernments, we cannot escape the all-too-frequent reality that enormous possibilities for removing risks of disease or death can be realized only at the cost of accepting or imposing other risks.

As James Childress and William Boley point out, then, Gustafson's framework for theocentric ethics requires "a form of consequentialism" in moral reasoning ([2], p. 393). Gustafson himself notes affinities between his approach and "classic utilitarianism" (in both its "act" and "rule" forms). Yet he also insists that, unlike utilitarian approaches, theocentric discernment can have "no single normative end or value" from which to assess probable consequences of various courses of action. While elements of utilitarian *procedures* are included in the process of discernment, that process also allows "discretion" in coming to a final perception of what is right and good. It must take into account, for example, such things as "right relations that serve the ordering of life, not only among human beings but also with nature." And because the considerations it must take into account are numerous and wide-ranging, theocentric discernment may arrive at an "ordering of priorities," but with no a priori certainty that the same abstract ordering is worthy of adherence in all situations ([16], pp. 112–14).

Now, of the three topical issues in medical ethics employed for purposes of comparison in this volume, nontherapeutic pediatric experimentation provides perhaps our clearest example of what Gustafson refers to as the most distinctive practical result of his theocentric ethics – namely, a greater emphasis on serving larger "wholes" than is to be found in many other prominent moral theories. Certainly that emphasis distinguishes his approach (and many of his conclusions) from those of McCormick, Ramsey or Hauerwas. Of course, that emphasis also requires an eschewal of the "anthropocentrism" Gustafson sees as rampant in contemporary ethics. And, frankly, our focus in this study has been limited to issues within the inescapably "anthropocentric" area of human biomedicine. Thus, our appreciation of the full differential scope of theocentric ethics must await Gustafson's further discernments on other, broader parts-vs.-wholes issues, such as the use of animals in medical experimentation, responsible forms of agricultural production, energy production/consumption and its ecological effects, etc.

The task of theocentric ethics – discerning, participating in, and relating all things in accordance with God's purposive ordering of creation – is not simple in any of its elements. As Gustafson is fond of reciting, from Milton's *Paradise Lost*, "So little knows / Any, but God alone, to value right / The good before him . . ." ([16], pp. 279–319, *passim*). Moreover, ethics from a theocentric perspective "does not guarantee us happiness, though it does not consign us to discontent" ([14], p. 342). But it does remind us, finally, that our desires and attempts to ignore or manipulate God, to "constrict" our perspectives and our loves to our own purposes, are simply the products of self-deception. For, ultimately,

God will not be manipulated.
God will not be ignored or denied.
God will be God ([16], p. 322).

NOTES

[1] For aspects of such "qualification," see [7], esp. Chapter 7.
[2] [17], p. 185. These thematic statements are drawn from Gustafson's 1981 Ryerson Lecture at the University of Chicago, entitled "Say Something Theological!"
[3] See, for example, [25]. See also David Schenck's response to some of Gustafson's critics in [30].
[4] [14], pp. 337–38. See also "Moral Discernment in Christian Life," in [6], esp. pp. 106 ff.

[5] [14], p. 338. Cf. Hauerwas's contrasting description of the phenomenon of moral choice in Chapter 4, above.
[6] [5], pp. 550–51. For a most cogent discussion of Gustafson's "casuistry" in this area, see [31].
[7] [5], p. 553. Gustafson never specifies exactly what he means by the evaluative term "ordinary" in this context.
[8] [16], p. 309. At another point, as if in response to Ramsey's insistence (following Kant) that we should never "use" research subjects or anyone else as mere "means" to another's ends, Gustafson points out that theological support can be given for "the instrumental value, the utility value" of persons: "If God is intent upon the preservation and cultivation of life, including as it must, men's lives in relation to each other and in relation to the rest of nature, a view of men as functionaries for the achievement of purposes consistent with those larger purposes is proper, and in order" ([4], p. 147).
[9] James Childress and William Boley, reflecting on Gustafson's argument that a "stringent adherence" to the rule of voluntary, informed consent could deprive many people of health benefits, note that, "as presented it opens the door not only to conscripting research subjects in order to save the larger whole of society in an emergency but also to produce various health benefits that would not otherwise be obtainable." And this is but one example of how Gustafson's part/whole approach qualifies traditional distinctions between moral obligation and 'supererogation' by "making many acts of self-sacrifice . . . obligatory, at least for theocentrists, in order to benefit the whole" ([2], pp. 393–94).

REFERENCES

1. Cahill, L.: 1985, 'Consent in Time of Affliction: The Ethics of a Circumspect Theist', *Journal of Religious Ethics* 13/1, 22–36.
2. Childress, J. and Boley, W.: 1987, 'Review of J. Gustafson, *Ethics from a Theocentric Perspective*, Vol. II', *The Journal of Religion* 67, 392–395.
3. Gustafson, J.: 1968, *Christ and the Moral Life*, Harper and Row, New York.
4. Gustafson, J.: 1971, *Christian Ethics and the Community*, The Pilgrim Press, Philadelphia.
5. Gustafson, J.: 1973, 'Mongolism, Parental Desires, and the Right to Life', *Perspectives in Biology and Medicine* 16/4, 529–557.
6. Gustafson, J.: 1974, *Theology and Christian Ethics*, United Church Press, Philadelphia.
7. Gustafson, J.: 1975, *Can Ethics Be Christian?*, University of Chicago Press, Chicago.
8. Gustafson, J.: 1975, *The Contributions of Theology to Medical Ethics*, Marquette University Press, Milwaukee.
9. Gustafson, J.: 1977, 'Interdependence, Finitude, and Sin: Reflections on Scarcity', *Journal of Religion* 57/2, 156–168.
10. Gustafson, J.: 1978, *Protestant and Roman Catholic Ethics: Prospects for Rapprochement*, University of Chicago Press, Chicago.
11. Gustafson, J.: 1978, 'Theology Confronts Technology and the Life Sciences', *Commonweal* 105 (June 16), 386–392.
12. Gustafson, J.: 1980, 'A Theocentric Interpretation of Life', *The Christian Century* 97, 754–760.
13. Gustafson, J.: 1980, 'Theology and Ethics: An Interpretation of the Agenda', in H. Engelhardt and D. Callahan (eds.), *Knowing and Valuing: The Search for Common Roots*, Institute of Society, Ethics and Life Sciences, Hastings-on-Hudson, N.Y., pp. 181–224.
14. Gustafson, J.: 1981, *Ethics From a Theocentric Perspective*, Vol. 1: *Theology and Ethics*, University of Chicago Press, Chicago.
15. Gustafson, J.: 1981, 'Ethics of Mechanical Ventilation', in C. Rattinborg and E. Via-

Reque (eds.), *Clinical Use of Mechanical Ventilation*, Year Book Medical Publishers, Chicago, pp. 340–46.
16. Gustafson, J.: 1984, *Ethics From a Theocentric Perspective*, Vol. 2: *Ethics and Theology*, University of Chicago Press, Chicago.
17. Gustafson, J.: 1985, 'A Response to Critics', *Journal of Religious Ethics* 13/2, 185–209.
18. Gustafson, J.: 1989, 'Roman Catholic and Protestant Interaction in Ethics: An Interpretation', *Theological Studies* 50, 44–69.
19. Gustafson, J.: 1990, 'Moral Discourse About Medicine: A Variety of Forms', *Journal of Medicine and Philosophy* 15, 125–42.
20. Gustafson, J.: 1993, 'Scientific Dreamers and Religious Speculation' (Review of M. Midgley, *Science as Salvation*), *The Christian Century* 110 (March 10), 269–274.
21. Gustafson, J. and Landau, R.: 1984, 'Death is Not the Enemy', *Journal of the American Medical Association* 252, 2458.
22. Hauerwas, S.: 1978, 'Can Ethics Be Theological?' (Review of J. Gustafson, *Protestant and Roman Catholic Ethics*, and P. Ramsey, *Ethics at the Edges of Life*, Hastings Center Report 8/5, 47–49
23. Hauerwas, S.: 1982, 'God the Measurer' (Review of J. Gustafson, *Ethics From a Theocentric Perspective*, Vol. 1), *Journal of Religion* 62, 402–411.
24. Hauerwas, S.: 1985, 'Time and History in Theological Ethics: The Work of James M. Gustafson', *Journal of Religious Ethics* 13/1, 3–21.
25. McCormick, R.: 1985, 'Gustafson's God: Who? What? Where? (Etc.)', *Journal of Religious Ethics* 13/1, 53–71.
26. McKenny, G.: 1993, 'A Qualified Bioethic: Particularity in James Gustafson and Stanley Hauerwas', *Journal of Medicine and Philosophy* 18, 511–529.
27. Outka, G.: 1983, 'Remarks on a Theological Program Instructed by Science' (Review of J. Gustafson, *Ethics From a Theocentric Perspective*, Vol. 1), *The Thomist* 47/4, 572–591.
28. Ramsey, P.: 1985, 'A Letter to James Gustafson', *Journal of Religious Ethics* 13/1, 71–100.
29. Reeder, J.: 1988, 'The Dependence of Ethics', in H. Beckley and C. Swezey (eds.), *James M. Gustafson's Theocentric Ethics: Interpretations and Assessments*, Mercer University Press, Macon, Georgia, pp. 119–37.
30. Schenck, D.: 1987, 'Prophecy, Polemic, and Piety: Reflections on Responses to Gustafson's *Ethics From a Theocentric Perspective*', *Journal of Religious Ethics* 15/1, 72–85.
31. Verhey, A.: 1993, 'On James M. Gustafson: Can Medical Ethics Be Christian?' in A. Verhey and S. Lammers (eds.), *Theological Voices in Medical Ethics*, Eerdmans, Grand Rapids, pp. 30–56.

CHAPTER SIX

SOME REFLECTIONS AND SUGGESTIONS

As the preceding chapters have illustrated, contemporary Christian theology manifests a variety of perspectives and approaches in medical ethics. The four moralists surveyed here differ among themselves not only in how they address and answer medico-moral questions but also in how they pose them. Their theological and anthropological presuppositions frame their views on the appropriate scope of ethical judgements (that is, whose interests or good must be included in formulating moral judgements), their understandings of the theological significance of human life and the experience of death, their selection of a preferred ethical methodology for resolving moral conflicts, and so on.

Some years ago James Gustafson advanced the thesis that any comprehensive and systematic account of theological ethics must have a central "discrimen" – an organizing perspective, principle, metaphor or analogy around which it is structured. That discrimen must relate in a coherent fashion four "base points": an understanding of God and God's purposes in relation to humans and the rest of creation; an interpretation of the significance of "the world" and human life in it; an interpretation of human moral agency and actions; and an interpretation of how we *ought* to make moral choices and judgements. Further, anyone who would construct and defend such an account must make judgements about its adequacy with reference to four sources: the historically identifiable sources of Christian thought (i.e., Scripture and subsequent tradition); philosophical methods, principles and insights; scientific information which is reasonably "solid" and relevant; and "human experience broadly conceived" ([7], Chapter 5). Now, elucidation of a theological ethics with systematic attention to all these base points and sources is certainly a tall order (and it should not be surprising that Gustafson's own account of "theocentric" ethics probably deals with them more comprehensively than do most other contemporary accounts of theological ethics). But I believe that even the rather cursory comparative expositions presented in the past four chapters have indicated very real differences among our four selected moralists regarding their prioritizations of sources and their "base point" interpretations. For brevity's sake I will not rehearse those differences source-by-source or base point-by-base point. But a couple of examples are perhaps in order here.

With respect to sources of theological-ethical insight, we can see a marked variety of emphases. McCormick gives primary emphasis to theological tradition – particularly the natural law tradition of a teleology of nature (and supernature) – supported by selected scriptural themes and modified by developments in the social sciences and historical human experiences. Ramsey's primary source is Scripture, but his "Protestant version" of natural law draws supporting evidences (of the human necessity of covenant fidelity) from human social experience. Hauerwas's major emphasis is upon the narratives of Scripture and Christian tradition through which we are enabled to interpret the realities of our experience. And, as we have seen, Gustafson's emphasis is upon the human experience of divine ordering powers, coupled with those scriptural and traditional symbols and concepts which can be consistent both with what we "sense" and otherwise experience and with evidences from the sciences. (The prominent interpretive/validational role given to the natural sciences is an aspect of Gustafson's approach which perhaps distinguishes his choice of source-emphases most·sharply from those of McCormick, Ramsey, or Hauerwas.)

Another, rather obvious area of contrast is the "base point" of preferred interpretations of how we should make moral choices and judgments. McCormick holds that we can and do perceive an objective order of values and that we should always choose to realize the highest or most basic available value (and/or avoid its destruction) in every moral choice, giving careful consideration to all foreseeable consequences of our choices. Ramsey, on the other hand, emphasizes strict observance of those general rules of practice which most fully express covenant fidelity toward each and every neighbor we confront. Hauerwas's primary emphasis is not upon dilemmatic moral choices at all, but rather upon the formation of moral character (and its attitudes, dispositions, etc.) through the narratives of a tradition, such that our descriptions of our situations and choices are truthful to reality as we have learned to envision it. Finally, Gustafson's ethical method is rather a balanced amalgam of value-centered, rule-centered, and character-centered approaches; certainly, however, his emphasis on the good of relevant "wholes" suggests that his model of moral discernment is more open to consequentialist reasoning than Ramsey's (or Hauerwas's) would be.

Now, if my understanding of what each of these moralists is trying to do is correct, at least for the most part, then what can be learned, for our own continuing theological-ethical reflection, from the juxtaposition and comparison of these four accounts of moral life? Seen together, what is their significance for the development of our moral perspectives and deliberations, other than to serve as interesting – and often conflicting – thought-experiments?

The answer, I believe – and the conviction that has made this comparative study worth the attempt – is that each of these Christian thinkers provides not only a fairly coherent and consistent alternative account of moral life but also provides useful nuances, adjustments, and even correctives to the other three accounts. Each reminds us of important perspectives and "points to consider" that the others have not emphasized. In some cases, one or more of their approaches may even provide bases for dealing with moral questions that cannot be fully addressed from within another of their accounts. (For example, Ramsey claims that a society's macroallocation decisions – that is, its selection of priorities for committing resources to broad social goods such as medical care, education, defense, etc. – are virtually "incorrigible to moral reasoning" – ([22], p. 240). This claim is not too surprising, given his insistence that our covenant-obligations toward individuals must not be overshadowed by calculations of collective goods. But I believe that moral frameworks for dealing with such macroallocation issues certainly are present in the approaches of McCormick, Hauerwas, and Gustafson.)

While there are, then, major differences (and even tensions) among the preferred models of moral choice and judgement we have surveyed here, I believe that our considered attention to these differences and tensions can and should be a source of moral discussion, growth, and enrichment rather than confusion. No single theory of moral being and/or doing can fully account for the ethical complexity of human experience. Value-based teleological theories, obligation-based deontologies, ethics of virtue and character, models of piety and discernment – all contribute important pieces of the puzzle, so to speak. Of course, any ethical theorist must have a starting-point, a primary model of moral judgement consistent with his/her sources of moral insight, understanding of human nature, etc., and around which relevant "points to consider" can be identified, organized, and weighed. In my own case, having been a student of much of the "teleology vs. deontology" debate in modern Anglo-American moral philosophy and theology, I have been greatly influenced by (and tend to think within the framework of) a deontological ethics of 'prima facie' duties. Yet I am also convinced of the wisdom in W.D. Ross's assertion that anyone who tries to work with obligation-based notions of the 'right' will inevitably be forced to deal with value-based notions of the 'good' as well ([23], p. 5). Further, notions of the right and the good do not appear to us from out of nowhere; we learn to recognize and interpret them, and develop attitudes and dispositions that favor them, through the formative webs of experience – or the stories, as Hauerwas puts it – of our traditions and communities. In addition – as Gustafson reminds us so forcefully – theological ethics must account for what we "sense" as well as how we "think." We cannot fully consent to our own beliefs and convictions if they are inconsistent with our affective experiences of reality and the "powers" we confront; nor could we ever fully recognize the "truthfulness" of inherited communal narratives without that affective confirmation.

In the final analysis, I believe that comparative study of the works of these Christian moralists can lead us not only to greater moral wisdom but also to a profound and necessary humility. And humility is a cardinal virtue for any theological understanding of morality. We are not God; we cannot see as God sees, we cannot value as God values. But we are nevertheless responsible for seeking, and orienting ourselves toward, God's will for us in our world and in our time. Whether we begin that search via an analysis of religious affections or the communal narratives which form our world-view, or by identifying particular values or obligations which seem implicit in what we can know of God's activity in the world, we must also recognize our own finitude and find ways of dealing with the moral ambiguities and tragedies we cannot avoid.

In a spirit of continuing the valuable conversations joined by these four moralists, then, I would like to suggest some of the theological-ethical directions in which I have been led through the reflective process of this investigation. These comments do not constitute any attempt at a systematic theology or ethics, but are offered as further reference-points in our ongoing dialogic search for theological truths and their moral manifestations. After presenting some general observations about the grounding and direction of Christian ethics, I will conclude by re-visiting the three medico-moral issues which have served as comparative examples in the previous chapters: competent patients' refusals of life-prolonging therapies; treatment decisions for seriously handicapped infants; and children's participation in non-therapeutic medical research.

1. CHRISTIAN ETHICS AS RESPONSE TO COVENANT PROMISE

To begin with, I believe Gustafson is quite right in his insistence that we give more attention to the profound significance of affective experience in religion and morality. 'Theology' cannot begin with abstract propositions about the qualities and characteristics of sacred powers, but instead must build toward such claims by reflecting upon our *senses* of divine power in the religious dimension of experience. And religious communication of experiences of the sacred depends upon the affectively evocative power of symbols, rituals, etc. Likewise, 'ethics,' as the reflective study of morality, cannot infer, deduce or posit normative claims about what is 'good' or 'virtuous' without affective experiential confirmation of their truth. 'Reason' can inform our sensibilities, yes, but reason alone cannot convince us to accept as positive that which we 'sense' in a profoundly negative way.

Moreover, it seems to me that any realistic answer to the question of fundamental moral motivation – Why *be* moral? – must be rooted in our senses of, and affective responses to, the realities we confront. There are, of course, a variety of possible answers because there are a variety of senses/responses which may dominate one's experience – *fear* of social or divine exclusion or punishment, *hope* for social or divine affirmation or reward, *anxiety* due to a sense of anomie or meaninglessness, or *defiance* against the sensed 'absurdity' of human existence, to name but a few. Certainly one of the most distinctive aspects of religiously-grounded moral perspectives lies exactly here:

in the motivation toward moral commitment grounded in the religious affections. Gustafson cites piety (awe and respect toward the sovereign Other) as the affective ground of "theocentric" ethics. And I would agree that such piety is central to any genuine theological-ethical understanding, at least in Western monotheistic religion. But I would add that in Christian piety the senses of awe and respect are suffused also with an overwhelming sense of *gratitude* toward the sovereign Other. That sense of gratitude – the primary affective ground of Christian moral motivation and commitment, in my view – is not evoked in some general way by the mere fact of our existence, and certainly not by any sense that our world is exactly as we would desire it to be. Rather, it emerges as our only possible response to the sense that we are forgiven, affirmed and made secure through God's covenant promise – the sense of promise that, as Paul wrote to the Roman Christians,

... neither death, nor life, nor angels, nor rulers, nor things present, nor things to come, nor powers, nor height, nor depth, nor anything else in all creation, will be able to separate us from the love of God in Christ Jesus our Lord (Rom. 8:38–39, *NRSV*).[1]

On an immediate, self-regarding level, such a sense of divine promise evokes our gratitude because it is a sense of personal security, of confidence that we will never be abandoned by the One who has power over all things. In addition, though, it evokes gratitude because it displaces or overwhelms any sense of anxiety that our lives and our world are without meaning or aim. And it assuages our fear of the unknown because it is a sense that the One who will never abandon us is also the Knower of all. As William May points out, our sense of God's covenant promise frees us from the fear-based need to avoid ties to those around us who are journeying into the unknown – the critically ill and dying – because they too are "no longer marked by the absence of God." Thus, in the arena of health care, for example, the sense of God's covenant promise allows for "a truly serious-light-hearted medical practice" ([16], p. 127f.).

As I see it, then, the 'story' of Christian being and doing begins with a moral motivation based not simply in a sense of God's awesome power but, more fundamentally, in a sense of gratitude for God's gracious and lasting promise. Further, I would suggest that this affective response of gratitude provides not only moral motivation but also a sense of *direction* for moral being and doing in the world. For, given that the sense of divine covenant promise is a sense of the reality of God's will or purpose for creation, then it would seem to follow, in my view, that the response evoked by it is not simply a generalized thankfulness but also a profound desire that this affirming, liberating perception of God's loving will should be realized and shared throughout the creation. This is, of course, the core of Christian evangelism, beginning with Jesus's 'great commission' to his disciples: to proclaim to the whole creation the reality of God's forgiving, reconciling love. And it is the core of Christian ethics exactly because it is the core of Christian evangelism. For, our experience of life in the world shows us that one's ability (or at least predilection) to sense anything like the covenant promise of God is a function not only of words heard but of the broader context of one's life-conditions (physical, emotional, spiritual, etc.) that limit, distort or enhance what can be experienced affectively in the first place. Thus, concern for 'proclamation' of God's covenant promise must also (or indeed, *first*) be concern for altering those life-conditions which may constitute barriers to its being heard and its reality sensed.

Dietrich Bonhoeffer, in his fragmentary and unfinished *Ethics*, expresses this point clearly, albeit in somewhat different terms. In one of his (several) attempts at identifying the foundations of Christian ethics, he argues that "penultimate" concerns (e.g., moral concerns about the welfare of others in the world) are important for the sake of the "ultimate" (i.e., "the coming of grace" or the "justification" of persons through the eyes of faith). "There are," he writes, "conditions of the heart, of life and of the world which impede the reception of grace in a special way, namely, by rendering faith infinitely difficult." Indeed, if a human life is deprived of "the conditions which are proper to it," then "the justification of such a life by grace and faith, if it is not rendered impossible, is at least seriously impeded." Thus, Christian morality involves removing those obstacles or barriers to others' experience of a sense of God's grace as a condition of the possibility of its proclamation to them: "The way must be made ready for the word. It is the word itself that demands it" ([4], pp. 134–37).

Now, if Christian ethics is viewed in terms of the covenant-response approach I am suggesting – as motivated by gratitude in response to a sense of covenant promise, and as directed toward removing obstacles to the possibility of that sense in others – then it becomes very difficult to isolate or draw lines between spheres of moral responsibility (e.g, 'personal' vs. 'social' ethics) or methods of ethical reflection (e.g., ethics of character vs. ethics of obligation; ethics of 'caring' vs. ethics of rights and duties, etc.). On the one hand, covenant-response is manifest in our very manner of life, our capacities for trust, encouragement and constancy, our ways of dealing with disappointments and tragedies, etc. – in short, our character. As Gustafson reminds us, persons do not experience the reality of God directly (except perhaps in rare cases of mystical transcendence or theophany), but rather indirectly, as the experience of something else. And while that "something else" may be a natural occurrence or historic event, it may also be the presence and life-model of another person (or community of persons). So, to put it bluntly, our manner of life may be either a facilitating means toward, or an obstacle to, the possibility of another's 'sense' of God's covenant promise. (Reflecting on my own experience, for example, I am aware that my sense of God's forgiveness, fidelity and unconditional love has been very much 'enabled' by my experience of those qualities in human terms, beginning in my parents' home.)[2] An ethic of covenant-response means, then, that (in Hauerwas-like language) our manner of life *is* our proclamation; in response to our sense of covenant promise we must live so as to enable response-ability to that promise in others.

On the other hand, though, I think it is clear that an ethic of covenant-response will also recommend, in both our personal choices/actions and our advocacy of social policies, adherence to those moral principles or norms which can be shown (based on our common experience) to promote "conditions proper to" a fulfilling life for others – conditions that may help facilitate a sense of "the coming of grace" in their experience. This would entail, too, a recognition of and respect for human 'rights,' not as exercises in tolerance but as reflections of the affirmative valuation of persons we sense in God's covenant promise.

This suggestion of the matter and manner of Christian ethics shares some significant "points of contact" with Ramsey's approach. I agree with him, for example, that the "main theme" of the biblical witness – and the most compelling theological base-point for Christian ethics – is God's covenant-faithfulness. And I would agree that our response to God's covenant promise could be described as "in-principled" (in terms of the sort of principles-adherence I have suggested above). At the same time, however, I do not believe that a covenant-response ethic can be manifest in a deontology as rigid as Ramsey's. The 'early' Ramsey (of *Basic Christian Ethics*) insisted that moral norms must be "derived *backward* by Christian love from what it apprehends to be the needs of others" ([19], p. 79). And this statement of the matter bears some similarity to my suggestion that norms be derived from our apprehension of what conditions might prepare the way for others' sense of divine covenant promise. Yet, as we saw in Chapter 3, Ramsey's understanding of covenant-response as "grateful *obedience*" led him to focus more and more upon its deontological character and upon his conviction that there are "some things that are as unconditionally wrong as love is unconditionally right" ([21], p. 129). Hence, many (if not most) of his later topical discussions emphasize his apprehension of what covenant-fidelity unconditionally (or almost-unconditionally) forbids.

While the covenant-response ethic I have described would certainly affirm that some things are at least presumptively wrong (i.e., can be shown to be barriers to "the coming of grace" in human experience, or tend to violate the basic conditions necessary for social interaction and cooperation), and while it would not deny the possibility that some things may even be always wrong, my central concern about Ramsey's approach has to do with his *derivation* of moral rules (including "exceptionless" rules), and particularly with his epistemic grounds for that process of derivation. He cites, as sources of moral wisdom, both the received biblical witness of God's covenant-faithfulness (and recorded human responses to it) and a phenomenology of covenantal relationships in human experience. Of the latter source – the core of his "Protestant view of the natural law" – he remarks that its content, its inherent meaning, is fulfilled in "the progressive discovery of new and relevant truth through unlimited discussion" ([20], p. 229). Thus, when he offers us the truths he has inferred or deduced about those choices/actions which clearly violate covenant-fidelity, I have to wonder *whose* "unlimited discussion" has yielded those truths, whose experiences of "covenant" verify his conclusions (and, of course, whether they will be sustained through "progressive discovery"). If his claims about what covenant-fidelity demands or forbids are intended to *provoke* "unlimited discussion," then Ramsey has been fairly successful in the attempt. But if he is claiming certitude about what will always be experienced by persons as manifestations or negations of covenant-fidelity, then I have to ask: Upon what evidence (cognitive and affective) and from within whose experience can such claims of certitude be made?

Of course, this question reflects a concern extending far beyond the details of Ramsey's particular approach, for it is a concern about the very 'arena' of moral discourse. Any account of ethics that depends upon what Gustafson calls "human experience broadly conceived" as a source of moral insight, interpretation and validation (as all of the accounts described in this volume do, to varying degrees)[3] must be concerned about the range or scope of human experience brought into moral dialogue. As I see it, an ethic of covenant-response must be, in a profound sense, an ethic of *listening* – particularly as it seeks to move from a broad, gratitude-informed directionality to more specific guides for moral life. And in that listening it must be attentive to a wide array of voices, past and present. It must listen to the voices of Scripture, those unparalleled accounts of the human struggle to discern and embody fitting responses to God's covenant promise; and it must listen to those voices we have from the faith tradition of persons and communities seeking to respond to their senses of covenant promise in a manner fitting for their life contexts. Further, however, because a covenant-response ethic is concerned to overcome obstacles to the human sense of God's covenant promise in our world, it must be able to discern where those obstacles lie. And that requires very active listening to the broadest possible range of voices among us, particularly those expressing experiential senses of despair, isolation, injustice and oppression in their life conditions. We cannot grant what God grants – we cannot bestow on others the sense of gracious promise to which we are responding. But insofar as that sense motivates us to "prepare the way for the coming of grace," as Bonhoeffer puts it, then it demands our attentiveness to those paths (and those obstacles) along "the way" which may lie outside the realm of our own immediate experience (both personal and communal). And as we listen to other voices of experience we must be ready and willing to reconsider our assumptions about those specific moral norms that will best embody, symbolize or express our gratitute and our desire to prepare the way for the coming of grace.

Now, these suggestions about Christian ethics as expressive of covenant-response are, I admit, rather tentative and sketchy. They do not describe a developed theory of morality to stand in contrast with the other four examined here, but rather a Christian perspective or affective stance from which to interpret our circumstances and respond to those around us. Yet, as I have tried to point out, such a stance does offer both a profound motivation for the task of moral discernment and a sense of direction in assessing moral aims and intentions.

With these suggestions as a starting-point, then, the final three sections of this chapter will consider the 'other end' of the ethical enterprise – namely, discernment and judgement regarding particular moral issues and conflicts. As I noted earlier, these commentaries are offered in a spirit of dialogue, as further contributions or "points to consider" within the conversations so ably advanced by McCormick, Ramsey, Hauerwas and Gustafson (and others). Thus, my reflections will often take the form of responses to particular thematic, metaphorical or deductive judgements advanced by them.

2. DECISIONS ABOUT PROLONGING OUR LIVES MEDICALLY: REFLECTIONS ON THE 'GIFT' OF LIFE

The issue of patients' refusals of life-prolonging treatment is one that can be viewed from a variety of interpretive stances, each with its own vocabulary. The vocabulary most familiar to contemporary Americans is that of rights-language – the hallmark of Western liberal political philosophy. Yet the notion of individual rights – and their justifiable limits – is in any case derived or inferred from other foundational concepts, such as 'natural' and essential human passions, tendencies and inclinations; the revealed commands of God; the *imago dei* in each person; etc. Each of the moralists surveyed in this study has tended to avoid any pronounced emphasis on rights-language in his discussion of treatment refusals; instead, each has focused upon particular themes, values, derived duties, and senses that can ground and limit our understanding of agential freedom in the medical treatment context. While their approaches (and their premises) have differed in many ways, all four[4] have appealed at some point to the theological metaphor of life as a *gift* from God, from which we may infer a duty of gratitude that limits in some way our understanding of agential freedom (or license) in choosing how or when to dispose of our lives. So, I believe it would be appropriate at this point to reconsider the metaphorical notion of life-as-gift and to offer a few suggestions about its applicability to the moral issue of autonomous treatment-refusals.

We should begin, I think, by considering our commonplace experience of the moral meaning of 'gift' – particularly in terms of the moral relationship established by it and the responses it invites or demands. For, any meaningful use of metaphor applied to divine-human interaction presupposes some familiar, accessible source of reference in our lived experience – in this case, our interpretation of 'gift' in human-human interactions. While it is probably true that commonplace definitions of 'gift' differ somewhat from time to time and place to place, the most persuasive paradigm definition with which I am familiar is that offered by Paul Camenisch [6]. He describes a gift as:

(1) some value (2) intentionally bestowed by a donor who gives it primarily to benefit the recipient upon (3) a recipient who (a) accepts it knowing that it is given as a gift, (b) agreeing with the donor that it is a benefit, (c) who has no right to or claim upon it and (d) who is not expected to pay for it in the future in any usual way . . . ; and (4) which brings into being a new moral relationship between recipient and donor, part of which consists of recipient obligations to the donor and the acceptance of limits upon the use of the gift ([6], p. 2).

In this understanding, a gift is not a windfall, a "boon from the blue" received without any knowledge of its cost to the donor or of the donor's present identity, motives or intentions, etc. On the other hand, neither is it a contractual transfer of value, a *quid pro quo* or negotiated trade or wage. Instead, a genuine gift creates (on the recipient's side) a relationship which is neither truly obligatory nor nonobligatory. We expect that one's willing acceptance of a gift evidences a sense or feeling of gratitude for the gift or for the donor's benevolent will; but that feeling is not true gratitude if the recipient also feels morally constrained or obligated to have that feeling! However, we also expect the willing recipient's grateful response to include "grateful conduct" toward the donor and "grateful use" of the gift. These aspects of grateful response fit more closely with our common-sense understanding of 'obligation'; yet a grateful response is more 'free' than most other obligation-responses in that the recipient is not strictly obligated to accept the gift and, if he/she does accept it, is generally seen to have some appropriate leeway and creativity in expressing grateful conduct and grateful use. Indeed, it is the freely-expressed nature of genuine gratitude which makes the gift-and-gratitude relationship morally richer than contractual relationships of specific rights and obligations ([6], pp. 8–11, 15, 21).

If Camenisch's analysis is true for our usual experience of gift and gratitude – and I believe it to be largely so – then what can we say about its theological application to God's willing donation of our lives, and our fitting response to that donation? Various Christian assertions of life's giftedness over the centuries have emphasized certain positive aspects of both gift and giver: that human life is a benefit we have not earned; that its giver intended our benefit in giving it, and thus we should be grateful to the giver for it; that the gift is still the giver's in some sense, so we should not wantonly abuse or destroy it; and that we should respond by being stewards or trustees of the gift of life and the manifold opportunities flowing from it ([6], p. 27).

However, there are significant conceptual difficulties in any attempt to describe our receipt of (and response to) our very existence in terms of other, more mundane experiences of gift-receipt and grateful response. The first and most obvious difficulty is logical (or perhaps metaphysical): In what sense can the 'gift' of one's own life be said to have a *recipient*? Unless we hold that a person somehow pre-exists his/her biological conception and birth, it makes no sense to speak of that person having *received* the (logically separate) *gift* of himself/herself ([13], p. 125f.). Perhaps a radical (and somewhat modified) Cartesian dualism of body/soul could make sense of such language; but most theologians who refer to life as a divine gift (including those surveyed in this study) clearly reject such a dualism. Ramsey's description of the human person as "an embodied soul or an ensouled body," for instance, leaves no room for considering oneself and one's mortal existence as separate entities.

Further, the notion of life-as-gift presents problems for any moral description of that gift-relationship. Even if I am able to conceive of myself as a recipient of the donated benefit of my existence, I may yet ask, How (and when) have I willingly *accepted* it as a gift? By the time one is able to understand any notion of life-as-gift he/she has been 'using' the gift for some time; yet such "inadvertent" acceptance of it cannot constitute the sort of consenting acceptance which normally grounds our moral expectation of gratitude and obligation on the recipient's part ([6], p. 28). And if we construct a notion of "presumed" consent to the gift, on what terms do we do so? Is consenting acceptance presumed to have been effective at some point in the agent's past, binding irrevocably for the duration of his/her 'natural' life span? Or is it, at the other extreme, presumed only until the agent is able fully to consent to receipt of the gift anew on a daily (or hourly) basis? Since we ordinarily hold that one who refuses a proffered gift does not thereby commit any moral wrong or sin toward the donor (although he/she may be forgoing future self-benefit in doing so), the question of whether a gift is willingly received is a morally significant one ([6], pp. 17–18). And convincing answers to it are not clearly evident in the context of one's consent to what (s)he already has or *is*!

This brings us to the question of morally appropriate *return* or other disposal of received gifts. When we find ourselves in possession of some unwanted or unneeded donation that we have not willingly accepted, Camenisch asks, "can we not return the gift . . . and so escape the recipient obligations?" ([6], p. 28). His implied affirmative answer is carried further by Eike-Henner Kluge, who insists that "a gift which we cannot refuse is not a gift; a gift which is not ours to dispose of is not a gift either, especially if we had no choice in accepting it" ([13], p. 125). Unlike other gifts in our experience, life itself cannot be returned or refused without also *destroying* it; it simply does not offer us the option of returning or rejecting (which involves no violation of recipient obligation) vs. destroying (which might be seen as insulting to the donor and/or others who recognize the value of the gift). Thus, it becomes all the more difficult conceptually to describe our very existence in the same way we describe other gifts. This difficulty, along with others cited here, has led Camenisch to conclude that "if life is a gift, it is so in a limited or a unique sense" ([6], p. 28).

Ramsey appeals to our moral sense of the ingratitude of gift-destruction when he avers that "choosing death" amounts to a "defeat" of God's gift-giving. Yet his further, highly polemical re-statement of the matter – i.e., that such a choice means "throw[ing] the gift back in the face of the giver" – would, with a different verb[!], describe a response which is not necessarily a cause for any moral offense. Return of a gift does not in itself bespeak any insult, ingratitude, or failure of obligation (although "throwing" it in the donor's face probably would). Ramsey's language implies that *any* deliberate choice for death (by a "non-dying" person) *must* invariably be seen, by metaphorical extension, not as a simple refusal or return of a gift but instead as the most insulting possible gift-destruction or gift-rejection. And in this I believe he has certainly over-extended his metaphor.

Of course, our moral assessment of the return of any gift must also take into account the recipient's *reasons* for returning it. If a particular gift should become painful or otherwise burdensome to its recipient, I do not believe we would judge that person's desire to return it as morally ungracious or a violation of obligation[5] – even if the gift had been willingly accepted at some point in the past. But that judgement would ordinarily rest in large part upon our sympathetic recognition of the recipient's claim that the gift had somehow made his/her *life* more difficult or unpleasant (and thus that return of the gift would allow for more beneficial life prospects). Is such a judgement (or its opposite) conceptually *possible* for us when the 'gift' in question is life itself, when its return may not only remove some of life's burdens (which we can recognize and understand) but will also result in an absence of all further mortal experience (to which we cannot relate at all)? Here again, we confront the difficulties inherent in attempts to view our lives as we do other 'gifts.'

Even so, some who employ the metaphor of life-as-gift allow that its burdensomeness may provide moral warrant for returning it (as with other gifts). Gustafson's treatment of suicide, for example, implies that our senses of gratitude, dependence, direction, etc., evoked by the powers that sustain us, are the bases for our construal of life as a gift. He goes on to say, however, that those powers may bear down upon a person in ways which evoke other, overwhelming senses, such that life is construed as an "unbearable burden" rather than gracious gift. And in such cases there may even be reason for "enmity" toward the giver of life as well as morally sufficient (albeit tragic) justification for choosing death. While I believe he is correct that some persons construe their lives as "unbearable burdens," I am not so convinced by his theological explanation of that construal. For, it seems to me that such a view of one's life (as opposed to seeing it as a 'gift') must have as its evocative source something other than some apparent caprice in the divine ordering of powers which, after all, also creates, sustains, governs and redeems all things.[6]

Gustafson's variable, sense-dependent construal of life-as-gift is not shared, of course, by McCormick, Ramsey or Hauerwas. But, for reasons adduced in this and previous chapters, I remain unconvinced by many of their applications of life-as-gift language as well. In fact, I suggest that, generally speaking, the gift metaphor itself is probably more confusing than useful when applied to the relationship between persons and their lives. For, we simply cannot relate to our cognitive and affective capacities, for example, as some separate entity, some *thing* we have received from outside the selves we are. Certainly I can interpret the *conditions* of my life, and things that happen to me, as 'gifts' added to my experience for which I am grateful. But that is true largely because I experience them as *relative* benefits (compared to other conditions or events I could imagine experiencing). I have no frame of reference, though, in which to assess my 'being' as a benefit that did not have to be but was nevertheless graciously bestowed upon "me."

Despite these reservations about describing individuals' own lives as divine gifts given to them, however, I believe that some descriptions of life as a 'gift' can be illuminative and compelling. For instance, Hauerwas insists that we should view our children as gifts. Seeing their lives in this way we realize that they are not simply products of our desires or objects of our creation; who they are and become is independent of our expectations. Further, they are educative gifts: they teach us "how to be"; they create in us "the proper need to want to love and regard another."[7]

Indeed, we might regard as 'gifts' the lives of all those around us whose presence sustains us and teaches us about how to love and regard others. For, from a perspective informed by a sense of God's covenant promise, they can be seen both as sharers in that promise and as symbols or expressions of its meaning in human form. Their presence and support enable and broaden our ability to sense God's constancy and love. Further, however, a sense of gratitude for God's donative promise (illuminated in and through those around us) impels us to *be* gifts to others, to become illuminators of the promise to which we respond. Thus, human relationships are, in a perspective of covenant-response, very much a matter of being-and-receiving 'gifts' of life.

In a similar vein, Hauerwas describes our role as 'gifts' to one another in terms of the narrative formation of selves. Our capacity for character, for attaining true "freedom," he writes, is a function of our ability to "see" our lives and our world truthfully, without self-deception. The narratives which give our lives meaning – and, more immediately, the claims upon us that force us out of self-absorption toward more truthful vision – come from others. Because of this, he says, our freedom is "literally in the hands of others." Without them we could not learn the stories that give our lives direction and purpose. In that respect, then, their lives are 'gifts' we could not do without. Likewise, our lives – particularly the stories we live out – are gifts to others. And part of the responsibility of *being* such a gift lies in affirming symbolically for others, through our attitudes and actions, the truths which our stories help us to see.

Now, my concern thus far has been to highlight conceptual difficulties in the life-as-gift metaphor's more traditional application and thus to focus upon a different, more relational understanding of it, rooted in a sense of and grateful response to the covenant promise of God. This interpretive shift, as I see it, also requires a re-orientation of the kinds of questions we raise for purposes of moral judgement in those cases where a person chooses against continuation of his/her life. I do not believe we should begin by asking whether (or claiming that) such a choice evidences a lack of gratitude on that person's part for the 'gift' of his/her being. Many different conditions, events and relationships in our lives evoke far more profound (because more experientially accessible) senses of 'giftedness,' and thus of responsive gratitude, than the mere facticity of our existence. And any sense of gratitude for one's life-situation is evoked differentially: quite frankly, some people have more to be grateful for in their lives than do others. As Bonhoeffer might put it, "the coming of grace" faces many more obstacles in some lives than in others. And this should give us pause before venturing to raise moral questions about the 'ingratitude' of anyone's decision to forgo further life among us.

Instead, I would argue that the Christian community's initial question in such a case should be, "How can we be gifts to this person; how can we live so as to embody for him/her our sense of covenant promise, security and hope?" That question is, after all, the demand of *our* gratitude. This does not mean that we should suspend all moral judgement of persons' desires and choices for death; we can and must make such judgements. But it means that we must first strive to create conditions that enable a sense of gratitude, hope and trust, that allow persons in pain or despair to envision and appreciate options in their lives other than simply ending them.

With these reflections in mind, then, let us turn to the particular issue of patients' refusals of life-prolonging treatment. Specifically, I want to focus upon situations in which competent individuals refuse means of medical aid that could extend their lives well into the foreseeable future (i.e., years or decades). Very few Christian ethicists would argue that incurable, terminally ill patients are morally obliged to accept whatever treatments will extend their lives (or, as some have put it, "prolong their dying") until all such treatments fail. As we have seen in previous chapters, however, there is more controversy over choices against continued life by those who are not clinically "dying" or even "terminally ill." How should we assess morally, and respond to, their decisions in favor of (relatively immediate) death?

One well-known case of this sort is that of Elizabeth Bouvia (described in Chapter 1). Her paralysis (due to cerebral palsy) and painful arthritis led her to consider her life not worth living; so she asked that her hygienic care and pain medication be continued but that she be allowed to refuse her feedings and starve to death. Another case, similar in many respects to Mrs. Bouvia's, made news in Michigan in 1989 ([26], [27]). David Rivlin, a 38 year old man, had been paralyzed since his spine was severed in a surfing accident 18 years previously. The degree of his paralysis had increased over the years to the point that he was quadriplegic, like Mrs. Bouvia. Unlike her, however, he had also been ventilator-dependent for two years. In the Spring of 1989 he requested that he be sedated into unconsciousness and then removed from the respirator and allowed to die. For, as he put it, "I can't see living like this for 20 more years. It's a barren existence. It's already a dead existence. It could turn a person bitter toward life and toward people, and I don't want that to happen to me." He had hoped "to have a family, a wife, children, a career, to be going places. None of that is going to happen. Ever" [27]. The nursing facility in which he resided refused to comply with his request, so he sought judicial relief. Because neither state nor county attorneys chose to contest his suit (to discontinue treatment), Oakland County Circuit Judge Hilda Gage refused to rule on it, except to state that all competent adults have a right to refuse treatment. So, Mr. Rivlin sought the aid of a physician willing to help carry out his wishes.[8]

In both of these cases, clinically "non-dying" patients – with life expectancies of at least 20 or 30 years – decided against medical prolongation of their lives. Now, some ethicists would no doubt argue that the cases are quite different, morally speaking, because the treatments at issue are fundamentally different. They might insist, for instance, that Mr. Rivlin actually chose against an unreasonably "burdensome" form of treatment (the respirator) whose employment had made his life disproportionately more miserable (albeit much longer), whereas Mrs. Bouvia chose *for death* by refusing nourishment which is not considered "burdensome" treatment but instead a necessary, beneficial part of everyday life. However, *neither* patient claimed to be seeking relief from burdensome treatment; both sought relief from *lives* burdened by intolerable (to them) physical conditions. Mr. Rivlin made clear that he hoped and expected he would not begin breathing on his own upon removal of the respirator, just as Mrs. Bouvia hoped and expected to die soon as a result of her fast. To that extent, then, both sought death as an end in itself or as a means of relief from physical and/or psychic torment.

I do not believe that the choice made in either case was an example of ingratitude on the patient's part. While I am grateful for the conditions and experiences of my own life, I have not lived as Mr. Rivlin or Mrs.

Bouvia have; I have not endured what they have endured. Given their circumstances, I cannot say that their decisions manifest any failure of grateful response.

Moreover, despite various anti-suicide interpretations of the scriptural commandment against murder (Exod. 20:13) since Augustine, there does not seem to be any explicit condemnation of self-chosen death in the biblical witness. Among the choices for suicide recounted in Scripture,[9] none are condemned (or praised) per se by biblical writers. King Saul, who fell on his own sword, is reported to have been accorded the same sacred annointment, burial and fasting rites as were given his three sons who died in battle (I Samuel 31:11–13). And Samson's self-chosen death, which accompanied an act of military retribution (Judges 16:23–31), is described as being *enabled* by the gift of superhuman strength he asked for and received from God. One rather popular line of explanation for several biblical suicides, dating back to Augustine, is that they were secretly commanded by God for divine purposes and thus were not fit subjects for human moral judgement. But such an interpretation amounts to some rather imaginative exegesis at best; or, at worst, profound eisegesis. In sum, it would be difficult to mount a convincing scriptural case against self-chosen death – at least in cases where one's life-situation involves great suffering and despair.

I would not argue that *all* choices for death via refusal of treatment are morally justifiable.[10] Some may be morally "frivolous," to borrow McCormick's language. But when a competent adult patient determines that medical sustenance of his/her diseased, injured or disfigured existence constitutes a personally intolerable burden, then I do not believe any of us have the moral or spiritual standing to judge that decision as ungrateful or cowardly. At the same time, however, those around that patient – family, friends, counselors, care-givers – have a tremendous opportunity and responsibility to *be* 'gifts,' to offer not only their sympathy and comfort but also their own glimpses of what makes life meaningful, to invite the one who suffers into their own 'story' of trust in divine sustenance, forgiveness and promise. This includes making known to the patient, in words and actions, that he/she is also a 'gift' to be appreciated and cared for.

Finally, our ministry to such patients should express appreciation for a shared aspect of the human condition that we might venture to cite as yet another 'gift': our capacity for free will and self-determination. It is certainly tragic when an ill or injured person decides that continued life is intolerable. But another sort of tragedy – perhaps a worse one – ensues when we respond by defeating that person's capacity to be himself/herself until the end (by denying his/her self-determination in favor of our own determinations). Moreover, interventions of this sort seem to me to smack of selective ingratitude – i.e., gratitude for (and expression of) our own free will without corresponding respect and appreciation of it in another. As I see it, persons contemplating death via treatment-refusal should be made aware of all realistic prospects for their future activities and abilities (including perhaps introducing them to others with similar afflictions) and should be offered every possible opportunity for involvement in decisions about their day-to-day care (for, after all, some may in fact be seeking death as an escape from a profound sense of powerlessness). However, when we are convinced that their decisions for death are informed and reasonably constant (as opposed to spontaneous), then we should not seek to supplant their considered judgments about the burdensomeness of their lives with our paternalistic judgements on their behalf.[11] In all of this, however, our efforts should be suffused with and express our sense that they, like us, are sustained in a web of divine care and concern that even death cannot break.

3. NEONATAL TREATMENT DECISIONS: MEDICAL INDICATIONS, PARENTAL AUTONOMY, DISTRIBUTIVE JUSTICE, AND THE BEST INTERESTS OF HANDICAPPED INFANTS

On August 2, 1988, five month old Samuel Linares aspirated a small balloon at a birthday party. By the time paramedics could remove the balloon from his windpipe Samuel was comatose due to brain damage caused by oxygen deprivation. He remained respirator-dependent in what was diagnosed as a "persistent vegetative state." After his parents were informed that he would never regain consciousness or breathe on his own, they asked that the respirator be removed and Samuel allowed to die. However, a lawyer for the hospital (which had no ethics consultant or Institutional Ethics Committee) feared that removal of Samuel's life-support might be construed as "child abuse" or "neglect" under the federal Child Abuse Amendments of 1984 [summarized in Chapter 1, above]. So the hospital refused to comply with the Linares' request unless they hired a lawyer and obtained a court order authorizing removal of the respirator – a process which would probably have cost them tens of thousands of dollars.

On December 23, 1988, Samuel's father, a $300-a-week laborer who already owed $200,000 for Samuel's care, attempted to disconnect his son's ventilator. He was wrestled to the floor by hospital guards. Later, on April 26, 1989, Mr. Linares unplugged the ventilator again, but this time he held the Neonatal ICU staff at bay with a large pistol. Samuel died in his father's arms ten minutes after his respirator was disconnected. Mr. Linares then surrendered the baby and the gun, saying, "I did it because I love my son and my wife."[12]

The case of Samuel Linares is both dramatic and tragic. I cannot condone the lengths to which his father went in order to allow his death; but neither can I find sufficient moral justification for the level of treatment Samuel received against his parents' wishes. His case is different from those of many other handicapped infants inasmuch as his medical condition resulted from an accident in infancy rather than from neonatal or perinatal illness or injury. Nevertheless, his treatment – like the treatment of so many infants with severe congenital anomalies – raises important questions about how we should assess the 'best interests' (medically and more generally) of imperiled infants, about the role and limits of parental autonomy (or "familial self-determination") in these matters, and about just distribution of the burdens and costs of intensive neonatal care. These questions will provide a framework for my reflections here.

Any ethical discussion of medical treatment choices for infants should begin, I believe, with the question, What course of action (or inaction) most accords with the child's best interests? For, if we believe (as I do) that all persons are created in the image of God and that our theological and moral significance as individuals is unique and non-quantifiable, then I believe it follows that our decisions (especially life-and-death decisions) on behalf of infants should be based upon what we can know or presume their interests to be. The problem, of course, is in discerning just what interests we can know or presume infants to have.

Ramsey's "medical indications" approach presumes that infants have a paramount interest in remaining alive via all useful medical means – at least until they are diagnosed as being irreversibly "in the dying process," at which point their primary interest shifts to the receipt of palliative or comfort care. This approach appears to have been followed closely by the drafters of the Child Abuse Amendments of 1984. As I noted in Chapter 3, however, a "medical indications" policy is not without conceptual difficulties. Can modern medicine discern with any reasonable certainty exactly when an infant enters the stage of irreversible "dying," or distinguish clearly between life-prolonging treatments and those which are merely prolonging the infant's dying process?[13] I see little reason for optimism in this regard.

Further, both Ramsey and the 1984 federal statutes stipulate that more-than-palliative treatment is not morally (or legally) required for infants who are "chronically and irreversibly comatose." (And I would assume that this category was intended by both Ramsey and the legislators to include infants in a persistent vegetative state, like Samuel Linares.)[14] But what is the *rationale* for such a stipulation? Are we to infer that life-prolonging treatment (beyond comfort care) is not "medically indicated" unless it can also restore a state of consciousness, or that the permanently unconscious infant no longer has a strong interest in having his/her life prolonged? In either case, we are still in need of some explanation as to why the child's state of consciousness makes such a profound difference, especially since the lives of many unconscious patients (of all ages) can be prolonged medically for months, years, and even decades.

The answer, I believe, is that these "medical indications" policies actually include a minimal "quality of life" criterion. Specifically, they assume that the (non-dying) infant's primary interest in continued life is conditional rather than categorical; it is conditional upon that life having the 'quality' of consciousness. Without the quality of consciousness, Ramsey tells us, the patient is "inaccessible" to our care (or, in other words, has no further interest in, and makes no claim upon us to provide, continued life-support). Consciousness is not the only quality Ramsey is willing to take into account, either. He states that some patients in "insurmountable pain" may be totally inaccessible to our care. And, as we saw in Chapter 3, he is sympathetic to the claim that life-prolonging treatments which themselves "diminish the patient's reception of care and comfort and a human presence" may not be in the (nondying) patient's best interests – a claim which involves consideration of the patient's prospective quality of life (if treatment is continued).

So, even approaches such as Ramsey's, which assess an infant's best interests according to "medical indications," generally include some sort of minimal quality of life criteria as well.[15] His vehement rejection of "quality of life" language actually amounts to an insistence that only certain sorts of quality of life criteria are morally relevant in assessing infants' best interests. He wants to be sure that non-patient-centered criteria, such as institutional inconvenience or familial and social prejudices and burdens, do not outweigh the patient's own interests. (This concern is shared by McCormick, Hauerwas, Gustafson, and this writer as well.) And the particular *measure* of patient-centered interests he employs is the patient's capacity or potential for *reception* of "care and comfort and a human presence." Interestingly, Ramsey's use of this standard is shared (though perhaps with a broader application) by Hauerwas and McCormick: Hauerwas suggests that handicapped infants may not have the moral interests and claims associated with being 'children' if their defects are so severe that there is "little possibility that they will ever be able to respond to care"; and McCormick cites "relational potential" as a measure of infants' interests in continued life. Insofar as our only reliable gauge of whether infants can *receive* "care" involves their ability to "respond" or "relate" in some fashion, there is a clear basis for kinship or commonality between these measures of infants' interests.

At the same time, however, McCormick's "relational potential" standard would measure not *only* the infant's capacity to "respond" to medical care but also his/her capacity (or potential capacity) for recognizing, and maintaining "meaningful relationships" with, those caring for him/her. Thus McCormick, unlike Ramsey, would be willing to say that some infants who are neither fully and permanently unconscious nor in "insurmountable pain"[16] may nevertheless have no profound interest in having their lives prolonged. This move away from consciousness and the absence of intractable pain alone as guidelines for moral judgement is shared, I believe, by Gustafson. For, while he does not offer specific guidelines for morally appropriate withholding/withdrawal of treatment, he does suggest certain "potentialities" which, if present, would indicate that the infant *does* have a strong interest in life-prolonging treatment. These include potentialities for "satisfaction in life," for fulfilling the infant's limited capacities, for "happiness," and for "providing the occasions of meaningful . . . experience for others."

Medical prognoses concerning these potentialities (or McCormick's "relational potential") cannot usually be made with as much confidence or specificity as can predictions of permanent unconsciousness or intractable pain (although even the latter are certainly subject to prognostic error). Moreover, any predictions about a handicapped infant's future "satisfaction" or "happiness" are subject to parents' or care-givers' valuations, based on their own experiences, of the meaning and requisites of satisfaction or happiness in life. We adults cannot know what a handicapped baby, who has never known what we call 'normalcy,' would find satisfaction in. And our attempts at making those discernments run the risk of involving us in what McCormick calls a "racism of the adult world." There are some good reasons, then, for holding that Ramsey's medical indications policy is not only practically simpler but also morally 'safer' than other, broader 'quality of life' approaches – safer in the sense that it involves relatively fewer opportunities for prognostic error or unjust discrimination against 'defective' infants based upon particular adult prejudices and presumptions.

Even so, I believe that a medical indications policy also carries with it a substantial risk – namely, a tendency toward unreflective vitalism, or a too-easy presumption that a handicapped infant's best interests begin and end with preserving whatever physiological functions he/she has remaining. Such a tendency would, in my view, place too little emphasis on the burdens (e.g., pain and isolation) an infant may have to bear in order to realize the medical 'benefit' of an existence which may be largely devoid of compensating human pleasures. Indeed, perhaps the most common criticism of a medical indications policy is that it mandates in some cases a violation of the Golden Rule, i.e., it requires that we subject babies to forms of treatment we would not be willing to endure ourselves (even presuming the best foreseeable outcome). And this concern should not simply be pushed aside because it involves the risk of judging our children's best interests according to our own prejudices. There are risks we must take, I believe, if we would seek to define those purposes and means of medical treatment which are most truly human – and humane.

Thus, I agree with McCormick that we should accept the responsibility (and the inherent risks) of making treatment choices for our children in ways which somehow reflect our understanding of what makes human life human. His "relational potential" criterion is, in my view, a reasonable beginning. I am not so certain as he is that all rational persons "prediscursively perceive" the essential good of sociality. But I would say, as a matter of empirical observation, that the prospect of permanent cognitive and relational isolation is extremely fearsome for most persons, and that human interrelatedness (or anticipation of it) is usually a precondition of our ability to wrest any genuine comfort – and certainly any meaning – from conditions of suffering due to pain or despair. In answer to those who would argue that the lack of relational potential does not itself cause the child any particular suffering, I would respond that it makes impossible the opposite of suffering, too. Without relationality one cannot *enjoy* the absence of pain or interpret the positive significance of pleasurable impulses, one cannot distinguish between satisfaction and simple endurance, and one cannot hope. Such an existence may retain the appearance and physiological functions of humanness, but it does not allow for the fulfillment of most human experiential 'interests.' It often does allow, however, for the negative experience of pain or discomfort. So I submit that infants with no relational potential retain a significant interest in avoiding pain, and our treatment choices for them should focus upon keeping them as pain-free as possible until they die.

Of course, handicapped infants who do have some relational potential also have an interest in avoiding pain and suffering. And I believe there are situations in which the painfulness of a child's condition or of particular treatments may be more than we could expect that child to have an interest in bearing, even for the benefit of prolonged life. True, we cannot *know* how much suffering an infant would be willing to bear for that benefit. But we do know that many (if not most) adults do not desire prolongation of their lives at any and all costs; and to assume that infants invariably would desire it may constitute another sort of "racism of the adult world."

To be sure, any judgement about whether continued treatment would be excessively burdensome for an infant is going to be an agonizing one, and one that should be considered with much circumspection and sensitivity to possible avenues of error. I would submit, for instance, that untreatable conditions of mental retardation, physical deformity or immobility should not be considered grossly burdensome to a baby unless they also entail extreme pain or discomfort. We should also bear in mind Hauerwas's caution that some suffering is an inextricable part of human experience, and thus should not simply be considered an 'enemy' to be destroyed even unto the destruction of the sufferer. Hauerwas is correct, I believe, that our efforts to avoid suffering for our children can become (and perhaps have become) obsessive. I agree with him, too, that the Christian story does not teach us to escape from suffering at all costs. I would add, though, that the traditional narratives of Christianity encourage us to bear up under our own sufferings while at the same time teaching us that God will not desert us and that we can have hope for the future. In other words, the Christian story offers us ways of interpreting our own suffering as purposive, sometimes even redemptive. That is what makes it humanly bearable. But can our understanding of divine assurance and hope make more bearable the sufferings of babies who will probably never be able to understand those sufferings as we do? Further, while this notion of accepting or tolerating suffering – whether our own or our children's – may be a strong argument against *killing* the sufferer for a quick end of suffering, I do not believe it necessarily means that we must enable or prolong a condition of suffering through medical technology. When life-prolonging treatment entails extreme pain or discomfort, or can only prolong a painful condition which will not become less so (especially when coupled with a prognosis of death in infancy or early childhood, as in the Tay-Sachs and Lesch-Nyhan cases mentioned in Chapter 3, or cases of Trisomy 13 or 18), then I believe it may (and often should) be withheld or withdrawn in favor of comfort care alone.[17]

Judgements of this sort require careful attention to all possible treatment options and prognostic possibilities in each individual case. There are some diagnostic categories (such as those just cited) for which the prognosis is relatively certain. But all too often – especially in cases of extreme prematurity – the possible success or futility of various modes of treatment, and the extent of their burdensomeness, can only be guessed at in the neonatal period. So I believe that, as a general rule, we should err on the side of caution (and of continued life) by instituting "medically indicated" treatment until its relative burdensomeness or futility can be more reliably ascertained. I admit that this approach could become *too* cautious (and thus not in the child's best interests) if it were combined with the sense of obligation some clinicians have toward continuing indefinitely all life-prolonging treatments once they have been instituted. But I would remind those who hold this view that withdrawal of a treatment which is no longer in the infant's best interests is morally no better or worse than withholding (not starting) that treatment on the same grounds. If the latter choice is morally justifiable, then so is the former.

These suggestions have been centered around substantive grounds or bases for discerning the interests that handicapped newborns may or may not have in life-prolonging treatment. But we must also ask *who* should have the primary responsibility for decision making on their behalf. It is clear that diagnostic and prognostic discernments, predictions about the pain and discomfort associated with various conditions and treatments, etc., are matters of clinical judgement. However, judgements about whether one would want to be kept alive under various conditions of non-relationality, pain, or discomfort are not clinical discernments but rather matters of personal valuation. Since infants cannot formulate or explain to us what their interests and values are, I believe that proxy decision making on their behalf should rest primarily in the hands of those most committed to discerning what the infant's best interests are and acting in accordance with those interests. And usually it is the parents who best fit that description. Now, some have argued that parents are not the most appropriate decision makers because they are not the most medically informed, impartial and disinterested parties.[18] And certainly some parents may be unable to comprehend the medical data given them or unwilling to place their baby's best interests ahead of their own psychological or financial concerns. On the other hand, though, our traditional understanding of 'family' includes the presumption that parents have shown an interest in their children's welfare by their willingness to bring them into the world, and that parents have a social responsibility to teach their children about the interests and values they should have. This is why our legal tradition has allowed parents so much discretion in decision making for their children in various aspects of life. Indeed, in many ways we expect parents to be anything but cooly "objective," "impartial," or "disinterested" in choosing what is best for their children. Families are, among other things, communities of shared religious and moral values, beliefs and expectations. So I submit that parental discretion should have a primary place in neonatal treatment decisions — at least where there is some reasonable basis for questioning whether continued treatment is indeed in the infant's best interests.

Of course, there have been (and will be) occasions of decisional conflict between parents and clinicians about what really is in a baby's best interests. If a physician believes that parents' wishes are not directed toward the child's welfare, then he/she has a responsibility to relate to them the bases of his/her disagreement (perhaps to the point of introducing them to others who have experienced similar predicaments). If the conflict persists, then either party should be able to consult an interdisciplinary body — an Institutional Ethics Committee or Neonatal ICU Ethics Committee — for review of the case and a hearing of both parties' positions and concerns. The role of the Ethics Committee is not, in my view, to adjudicate but rather to facilitate exploration and analysis of available options and their ethical rationales. However, if the committee concludes that the parents' wishes do not comport with the infant's best interests, then I believe that conclusion should be shared with the hospital administration, which could then seek judicial review of the case. In any event, the parents should be treated from the outset not as adversaries or outsiders but as persons who are assumed to care deeply for their children and who are in need of personal support as they share in their baby's suffering.

Sadly, not all parents are willing to put their infant's best interests first in neonatal treatment decisions. And medical care-givers (and society in general) have a responsibility to try to protect the infant's interests through the sort of procedural mechanisms I have noted here. At the same time, however, I would venture to say that the federal government has gone too far in attempting to restrict parental (and clinical) judgement. As the reader is certainly aware by now, my approach to assessing a defective infant's best interests is not quite so narrow as that of the Child Abuse Amendments of 1984. Indeed, I believe there may be occasions in which "conscientious objection" to the apparent statutory requirements of the law may be morally appropriate (for parents, clinicians, hospitals, and even state legislatures). For I believe that some instances of life-prolonging treatment may be morally unreasonable or "inhumane" even if they do not appear to meet the statutory definitions of "futile" or "virtually futile" treatment. Further, I suspect that in most cases an infant's best interests can be sufficiently protected without such statutory stipulations if the "publicity test" (to use Sissela Bok's term) afforded by an informed and thoughtful Institutional Ethics Committee is made available. (And even with the 1984 statutes in place, I believe that the input of an IEC could have avoided the tragic denouement of the Samuel Linares case.)

Now, as a final area of consideration in this section, I believe we should reflect upon the *costs* of intensive infant care and the distribution of those costs. This is an issue which has been virtually pushed aside in many discussions of neonatal treatment decisions, probably because it tends to invite utilitarian-sounding cost-benefit or cost-effectiveness analyses that threaten to overshadow our concern for the best interests of infants themselves. But the ever-increasing expense of life-prolonging medical technologies has forced major industrial nations into a new era of soul-searching about who will receive these expensive forms of care, on what grounds those allocations will be made, and who will pay for them. Neonatal intensive care is one of the most expensive (per patient) arenas of modern health care delivery. And it would not be surprising if cost concerns were identified as the most common extrinsic (i.e., non-patient-centered) factor in parents' decisions against maximal treatment of severely handicapped infants. After all, parents cannot simply ignore the present and future economic needs of their other children and themselves.

One of the most common criticisms of the 1984 Child Abuse Amendments was that the new regulations not only mandated treatment choices which parents may not believe to be in their babies' best interests but did so within a context of shrinking federal funding for the provision of those treatments. Put in other words, the government was demonstrating a decreasing willingness to enable the forms of care it was requiring. This criticism points, in my view, to the broader question of the relationship between parental and societal responsibilities for furthering children's welfare in light of parental and societal authorities for defining their welfare. And any possible answer to that question, as Hauerwas would remind us, must be premised in large part upon some shared understanding of the meaning of 'family' and 'parenting.' If we envisioned the family as an isolated moral and social entity, self-legislating and responsible only to and for itself, then we would have little reason ever to question or challenge the decisional authority of parents in matters relating to their children; also, parents would be expected to provide the wherewithal to effect whatever choices they make.

But that understanding of family has never issued from the narratives of the Hebrew or Christian traditions. Instead, we have come to see parental authority and responsibilities as grounded in the interests and values expressed by, and expectations formed within, the communities in which families exist. I believe Hauerwas is largely correct that to be a parent is to "perform an office for a community of seeing that a child finds his or her way to the moral best that the community has to offer." If this is so, it means that parents who are seeking to promote their children's best interests (as those interests are communally understood) are also promoting the community's interests. The welfare of children is a value to the community as well as to parents. It follows, I think, that the community has a responsibility to help enable the promotion of infants' best interests. This is particularly crucial when parents are not financially able to do so on their own. Certainly parents should be the primary guarantors of the means to their children's well-being; but they should not be expected to bear catastrophic medical costs alone. A community should be willing to put its funds where its proclaimed interests are.

Another way of stating this is that handicapped infants in need of expensive medical treatment should not be discriminated against on the basis of their parents' inability to pay. It is true, of course, that ability-to-pay has always been a factor – often the deciding factor – in the 'rationing' of health care delivery in the U.S. That is one of the moral failures of our society, in my estimation. But even a society unwilling to discriminate on that basis faces difficult allocation questions in most areas of health care delivery, including neonatal intensive care. No society is able to provide all the resources needed by all of its members on a constant basis. Value-judgements must be made as to the relative funding priorities given to very different human needs (e.g., national defense, education, housing, proper nutrition, medical care, the arts, etc.). As I see it, the just society is one which gives priority to meeting the most basic human needs for all. That priority would, I believe, most clearly embody a grateful response to God's covenant promise by seeking to promote conditions that enable "the coming of grace" in human life. And that priority would certainly mean a strong emphasis upon access to health care for all. However, even the allocation of huge resources to the health care arena (at the expense of other social goods) may not guarantee the availability of all 'indicated' technologies for all who need them. Medical resource rationing can be necessary not only because of the limits set by broader allocation decisions but also because of other non-monetary limitations – e.g., the limited number of organs available for transplantation, shortages of new drugs derived from naturally scarce materials, or even staffing or bed limitations in a given facility. All of these limitations – and many more – are presently facts of life in the American health care system. Our question is not *whether* to ration but rather *how* to ration justly.

I do not intend to analyze or defend a range of rationing options here; that would require another lengthy study. But, in the particular area of neonatal treatment decisions, I believe that at least one sort of rationing approach emerges from the above discussion of handicapped newborns' best interests. Specifically, in cases where a baby's illness or handicaps are so severe as to preclude an interest in life-prolonging technologies, provision of those expensive treatments may be something less than morally 'optional' – it may indeed constitute an unjust allocation of costly medical resources. I would argue that none of us has a clear 'right' to treatment that is obviously futile, especially in a context of limited resources for all. Thus I believe a society may justly ration its neonatal care resources by 'discriminating' against futile forms of treatment. Further, infants who cannot attain consciousness or relationality (such as Samuel Linares) have a claim for the provision of appropriate comfort care (particularly amelioration of any painful sensations), but are not treated unjustly if they are denied further life-prolonging treatments such as ventilators, renal dialysis, intravenous nutrition/hydration, etc. Some parents who can afford maximal life-prolonging measures may choose to provide it, and perhaps that should not be discouraged – at least not yet (although I also believe that aggressive treatment in some cases can be unjustifiably *cruel* as well as expensive). However, I believe that communities and governments (and at some point perhaps even private insurers) that cannot afford to meet all medical needs should begin any necessary rationing of neonatal treatment technologies by forgoing them for those who have the least genuine human interests in them. Such rationing may indeed become a necessary precondition of our ability to provide costly life-prolonging care to those infants who *do* have a tremendous interest in it. The case of Samuel Linares, for instance, would have been even more tragic if his lengthy presence in a NICU had limited the staffing, space, or technological resources necessary to save the life of another baby with a hopeful prognosis.

Any form of rationing will be painful for some persons, and the present suggestion is no exception. Parents who cannot afford costly life-prolonging treatment in the sorts of cases cited here may nevertheless feel a profound sense of obligation to "do everything" as an expression of their commitment, and they will surely be anguished if that choice is denied them. In a very real sense, their interest in symbolizing parental love and concern is sacrificed in order to increase some other children's chances for a healthy life. While that is tragic and a cause for regret, I believe it is less damaging to both individual goods and the common good than other, perhaps inevitable forms of rationing might be.

Now, nothing in the foregoing discussion is meant to imply that treatment decisions for grossly handicapped, poor-prognosis babies can be made easy or clear-cut. They cannot be. But such decisions should and must be made carefully, with the best available diagnostic and prognostic advice, with primary emphasis upon those human interests which may yet be present or possible for the infant, with due consideration for parental authority and responsibility, and with concern for the distributive justice questions raised by intensive treatment of those who may not benefit from it.

4. CHILDREN IN NONTHERAPEUTIC RESEARCH: COVENANTS, GRATEFUL RESPONSES, AND THE INTERESTS OF CHILDREN

The four moralists surveyed in this study have taken markedly different positions on the issue of nontherapeutic research involving children, ranging from Ramsey's flat rejection of it to Gustafson's apparent justification of more-than-minimal subject risk in some circumstances. The variety of their conclusions is not surprising given the diversity of their thematic starting-points: duties of social justice derived from natural tendencies toward sociality; exceptionless rules expressing "covenant faithfulness" in research relationships; the moral meanings of 'child' and 'medical progress' within a community's narrative understanding of itself; and our shared responsibility for the flourishing of various "wholes" in creation. In what follows here I will reflect, selectively, on a few of the arguments considered in previous chapters (and elsewhere) and offer some constructive suggestions on the issue of pediatric experimentation.

I will begin with Ramsey's notion of covenant faithfulness. For, I do believe that God's covenant faithfulness provides a central focus for our interpretation of the biblical witness. And I would agree that we also discern something of the moral reality and necessity of covenant fidelity in our experiences of human social relationships. But I am not at all certain that our covenant responses are best expressed in a rule prohibiting all nontherapeutic pediatric research. There are, I think, significant aspects or dimensions of our experiences of covenant that are absent or undeveloped in Ramsey's analysis. In general, his description of covenantal responsibilities in medicine and research is notably uni-directional and individualistic; his concern is almost exclusively with the nature and limits of professional obligations toward patients/subjects. He virtually dismisses the idea that research subjects may have any covenantal responsibility to be research subjects by insisting that all medical experimentation for the benefit of others be understood simply as a matter of optional, voluntaristic "charity." I wonder, though, whether such a view can be maintained so decisively if the enterprise of medical research is viewed in a context of broader covenantal relations and responses within and among communities and generations.

We experience social covenants in many different forms, and in some of them our participation and covenantal responses – and even those of our children – are expected or implied rather than being matters of explicit "consents." The family is perhaps the best example of this: small children are expected to participate in activities which promise no particular individual benefit for them but which nevertheless symbolize and express the family's unity and interdependence. As Gustafson might put it, we expect their positive responses to certain claims made upon them by relevant "wholes" in which their interdependence with others is manifest. Somewhere down the spectrum of social covenants we might also point to the example of individuals' relationships with the State. The purposes of government in this country (common defense, maintenance of individual freedoms, provision of public education and some other forms of welfare assistance, etc.) are supported through taxation; and we have come to expect that all those with a certain level of wealth or income, regardless of their age or mental development, are expected to participate in that support even though they may not benefit individually from many of government's policies and programs.

Could we make sense of a notion of "implied" covenant and covenant-response among generations of research subjects and their beneficiaries? I believe so – at least in some limited form. We are all beneficiaries of past medical research developments. Others have borne the risks or inconveniences of experimentation that allow us opportunities for healthier lives. Their activities might be seen as part of the initiation of a covenantal promise, a promise that new avenues of medical aid to those in need of it will not be ignored but instead understood as opportunities for our common flourishing. And that promise is also an *invitation* for our covenant-response. For, the advancements of medical research produce not only answers but also new questions, new possibilities for flourishing that remain to be tested. And we, for whom the promise of research has been so richly kept thus far, are invited to keep it alive and growing for our generation and those to come. Certainly we have the freedom to decline that invitation; but is that a morally appropriate response?

Obviously, this question pushes us to consider once again the moral implications of *gratitude* – in this case, gratitude for a beneficial promise made and kept. While some would argue that human social covenants are virtually "contractual" in nature, and thus evoke something other than "grateful response," I believe that gratitude is at the very heart of many of our experiences of "covenant" – especially, e.g., marital and familial covenants. (And, of course, a theological understanding of biblical models of covenant involves notions of promise, invitation, and expectation of grateful response. The Exodus, for example, and the "new covenant" given in Jesus Christ, are hardly contractual arrangements; they are promises made and kept which invite grateful human response.)

It would not be inappropriate, in my view, to refer to contemporary medical cures and treatments as 'gifts' that enrich our lives – gifts promised and delivered to us by past researchers and subjects, to whom we owe gratitude. And, as I have already suggested, our most appropriate expression of grateful response would be acceptance of their covenantal invitation to keep alive the promise of human flourishing through continued medical research. Now, such a suggestion would be criticized by moralists such as Paul Ramsey and Hans Jonas, who insist that our gratitude is owed to past research subjects as individuals and, moreover, cannot be the basis of any social *obligation* of further research participation on our part. As Jonas puts it, "gratitude is not an enforceable social obligation; it anyway does not mean that I must emulate the deed" ([12], p. 15). Jonas may be correct that our gratitude for past research efforts does not entail that we *must* "emulate the deed"; but what I am suggesting is that such emulation is perhaps the most appropriate expression of grateful response. And I would agree with him that, generally speaking, gratitude is not an "enforceable social obligation." I would never argue that it is, or that anyone should be forced into research participation against their express will. But there are moral attitudes and responses – gratitude among them – which we often *expect* or *presume* of persons (unless their words or deeds indicate a different direction) even though we would not think of *forcing* their expression. And besides, I do not believe that the central moral question regarding (proxy consents for) nontherapeutic pediatric research is "Should we *force* this on our children?" anyway. Rather, it is a question of whether parents should be allowed to express, on their children's behalf, the covenant-responses they expect, presume or hope for in them. My comments here are meant to suggest that there are good moral reasons, grounded in gratitude to and covenant fidelity with past research subjects, for at least an initial presumption that present beneficiaries of medical advances, including children, would not object to furthering those advances through their own (minimal-risk) research participation.

I should point out that this approach is substantially different from McCormick's. He seeks to establish a (limited) moral obligation of research participation as a matter of social justice. His grounds for that obligation are, first, our natural inclination toward the good of "sociality" (through which we recognize that our own flourishing is interconnected with the well-being of others), and, second, the fairness of "bearing our share" of the research burden if we expect to share in the advances resulting from it. While I am inclined to be sympathetic toward his fairness argument, my focus here is upon the sort of "grateful response" we might expect of each other rather than upon our duties of justice to one another. To the extent that grateful response can be called a moral "obligation" at all, it is certainly a less stringent (and less "enforceable") obligation than are our duties of social justice. Yet that does not diminish its significance as a basis for our moral expectations and judgements. The "initial presumption" I have outlined here is in part an application of the more general negative claim that we do not expect persons to be ungrateful for benefits they enjoy as beneficences from others.

Such a presumption is, of course, only a presumption; it cannot and should not be used to override the objections of those who choose not to consent to research participation. But it might provide a significant starting-point for our consideration of proxy or surrogate consents on behalf of those whose own willingness or unwillingness to consent cannot be known explicitly – i.e., children and other incompetent persons. And the question of proxy consents for children – particularly the question, "What would this child want if he/she could tell us?" – has been such a difficult one precisely because any answers we might offer must be based upon our own presumptions of one sort or another.

In this regard, Ramsey's version of what we can presume offers a relatively simple solution. The only thing we can observe empirically about the wishes of infants and small children, he tells us, is that they are inclined toward self-preservation and healthy life and growth for themselves. Thus we may presume that they may want the prospective medical good (for themselves) afforded by participation in therapeutic research. But they exhibit no apparent inclination toward benefiting others, so we cannot presume that they would want to participate in nontherapeutic research. This assessment of what we can and cannot presume about children's desires has the virtue of protecting their interests from the possible results of various other presumptions about them (e.g., that they would be willing to consent to experiments with high subject-risks if the prospective benefits to others were even greater). It is intended, in fact, to isolate or protect children from the 'adult' world of moral claims and expectations. But to what extent is such isolation really what we want for our children? To what extent is it even in *their* best interests, all things considered? If Hauerwas is correct that parents have a responsibility to "initiate their children into the best form of life they know" ([10], p. 132), and if that form of life includes at least minimal expectations of grateful response and some sense of fidelity toward one's peers (as I believe it does), then why should we also presume (as Ramsey does) that children, if they could express themselves, would want no part of that life – at least not yet?

None of us can know for sure what small children do in fact want for themselves or others; we cannot know which of our presumptions on their behalf may be accurate. In the case of previously-competent adults who are now incompetent, we can look to their past expressions of interests and desires as guidelines for what their present choices might look like. But small children have no real 'past' as valuing, decisional agents; they are not-yet-agents, or perhaps agents-in-becoming. So, any attempts to specify what an individual child "*would* want" are essentially *proleptic* in the sense that they are claims about how a child would formulate and express his desires and responses *if* (s)he already possessed those requisite interpretive and decisional skills which are in fact not yet developed. And this presents rather obvious conceptual problems.

One possible resolution would be to refrain from *any* attempt to specify what our children's interests and responses would be until they are capable of expressing them on their own. Another would be Ramsey's approach: to specify only those interests and responses we believe we can infer from our empirical observation of children's behavior. A third approach (which I favor) would, like the first, refrain from speculation about what small children *do* seek as individuals. But it would self-consciously replace some of that speculation with *anticipation* of what we hope and expect our children *will* want (and will even approve of retrospectively for themselves) as they are initiated into the best form of life we know. This approach is admittedly paternalistic (or maternalistic): it involves making certain choices for children now because we anticipate that they will 'ratify' those choices later – not when they become 'rational agents' per se but when they become the sort of persons we are trying to teach them to be. Now, I realize that this sounds not only paternalistic but also deterministic; and it is, to some extent. For, it recognizes the reality that children do not and cannot become 'agents' in a moral or spiritual vacuum; they cannot simply step into their agency untouched and unformed by "deterministic" influences of parents and others within their communities. As Hauerwas bluntly states, "[o]n important matters children simply do not have interests until they have been taught what interests to have" ([10], p. 133). Some interests, such as avoidance of harms to oneself, are learned more quickly than others; but I think it is reasonable to claim that we presume a variety of interests on our children's behalf in anticipation of their learning them and consciously affirming them in their characters.

Something of the spirit of this approach to discerning what children "would want" is implicit, I believe, in a proposal submitted by William Bartholome to the National Commission for the Protection of Human Subjects [1]. Bartholome takes issue with Ramsey's assertion that children have no interest in nontherapeutic research participation because it offers no clear benefit to their own growth and flourishing. While it does not offer any *medical* benefit to them, Bartholome counters, it can and may provide an opportunity for their "moral growth":

> ... In order that children might become sensitive to moral obligations and develop a disposition toward choosing that which is good, they must experience situations in which that sensitivity is required and which enhance this disposition. I would argue that involvement in 'no risk' clinical research *can* be such an experience ... ([1], p. 3.17).

Bartholome goes on to deny McCormick's contention that we all have an obligation of social justice to participate in such research. So, the moral sensitivity and "disposition" to which he refers may relate, I think, to a moral sense of gratitude and a disposition toward covenant-response as I have described it. It seems, at least, that he is looking toward the outcome of what interests we are trying to teach our children to have as a basis for presuming those interests on their behalf in the here and now. And I believe his presumption is reasonable.

Bartholome goes on to insist, further, that if a child's moral development is the rationale for our presumption of his/her consent to research participation, then the conditions of that participation must be fully conducive to moral education. And in his view this means that the child must be old enough (at least 5 years of age) to understand the experiment's purposes and procedures and to agree to them. Also, he says, the parents should act as moral examples by participating in the experiment themselves – as co-subjects when that is realistically possible, or in some sort of supervisory capacity at the very least.

I would agree with Bartholome that parents should be involved somehow along with their children, not just because they should be moral models for them but also because their choices should express (symbolically and practically) the very interests they presume on their children's behalf. Any parent unwilling to recognize and accept a covenantal invitation to participate in the promise of medical progress has no reason to expect that his/her child would (or will) accept that invitation.

At the same time, however, I do not agree fully with Bartholome's requirement that children must be excluded from nontherapeutic research participation until they are old enough to understand its purposes and agree to it. His rationale for this requirement may be that he considers his own model of presumed consent to be a mere pre-condition for legitimate proxy consent – a pre-condition that must be supplemented by some reasonable facsimile of the child's *actual* consent in the form of his/her present "assent." I suspect, though, that his real rationale has to do with what he considers the practical limitations of moral education – namely, that a child cannot learn much about the moral significance of research participation unless he/she understands and accepts what is happening at the time. This is probably true in the negative sense that a child who *disagrees* but is nevertheless dragged kicking and screaming into a research protocol is unlikely to learn much about his/her moral interest in research participation. Thus I believe that children who show evidence of understanding the particulars of a research protocol should be allowed opportunity to dissent and should have their dissents respected. After all, any presumed or imputed interest they may have in expressing gratitude or fidelity would be outweighed by their presently-expressible interest in avoiding what they consider overly fearsome or painful.

But this consideration presupposes that the research protocol in question may be of a sort that children would indeed consider fearsome or painful. I submit, then, that our first concern about any protocol should be with *why* a child might dissent rather than with the mere possibility *that* he/she may dissent. We should never presume consent or seek proxy consent for children's participation in nontherapeutic research if we have reason to believe that particular child-subjects (or children of that age in general) would find the protocol hurtful or otherwise frightening. Now, discernments of this sort are, admittedly, not always easy. And they must be particularized to some extent, for some children are frightened by environments and experiences that are not at all threatening to others (Ramsey's "empirical" approach to discerning what children would want may be useful in this regard, since parents and others who work with children have many opportunities to observe fearful reactions in various contexts). I would suggest, at least, that small children (and even children older than Bartholome's 5-year minimum) should never be expected (or asked) to undergo invasive, risky or probably-painful research procedures (e.g., venipuncture or urinary catheterization) – unless that procedure is already required for some other therapeutic or diagnostic reason.

Because my emphasis here is upon what a child might *object to* rather than upon whether the child is fully able to give an understanding "consent" (and I have my doubts about Bartholome's age-related standard for the latter), and because I believe we can have a pretty good idea about what even very small children might object to, my approach to the proxy consent issue would not follow Bartholome's in automatically ruling out research participation for children younger than five years. For, I do not share his implied premise that research participation cannot be morally educative or formative unless the child understands and is able to assent to it beforehand. Young children are often involved by their parents in activities whose meaning or significance they are not expected to understand until later. And I see no reason why the activity of research participation could not provide a valuable basis for moral education (through recollection and reflection) as children develop the capacity to comprehend its meaning. (In this regard, I suggest that all child-subjects should receive a final written report of their research protocol's purposes, results and medical significance for their later examination and reflection.)

I realize that this approach to proxy consent leaves open a somewhat greater range of possible mistakes or abuses (that is, choices based upon something other than the child's presumed interests and non-dissent) than does Bartholome's. For we cannot read the minds and hearts of parents who offer proxy consents. At the same time, however, other standards of 'consent' are not immune to mistake or abuse, either: we cannot be absolutely certain about the fully "voluntary" and "informed" nature of many *actual* consents by mature minors and adults.[19]

Further, it is frequently pointed out that the research data necessary for medical advances beneficial to small children often cannot be obtained at all except through the research participation of young child-subjects. And this reality might (as Ramsey argues) create for some a strong temptation to 'weigh,' in utilitarian fashion, potential subject-risks against potential therapeutic benefits for other children. Yet I believe we can (and must) draw a line against or contain that temptation by simply ruling out any significant potential subject-risks at the outset. In other words, we must make every effort to insure that nontherapeutic pediatric research protocols would not be risky (or painful or frightening) to small children *before* their parents' consent is ever sought. Institutional Review Boards overseeing pediatric research have a special responsibility to be sensitive in this regard. Such IRBs should,

I think, include among their members specialists in child psychology and development, and perhaps also parents of small children from the surrounding community. After (and only after) the IRB has carefully examined a given protocol's procedures and has deemed them non-risky and non-threatening to children (of the potential subjects' ages) in general, then I believe it may be reasonable to accept proxy consents from parents who believe their children would not dissent and who expect that their children will come to share their (the parents') interest in responding positively to the covenantal invitation afforded by nontherapeutic research's promise of benefit for other children.

Now, this discussion has been centered around the question of proxy consent in nontherapeutic pediatric experimentation, largely because that question has been the focus of so much analysis and critical conversation heretofore. Yet it is not, of course, the only matter of moral judgement requiring our considered attention in this area of medical research. (I have argued, for example, that proxy consent should not be sought or invited until it is clear that the protocol will not involve any significant foreseeable risks for its subjects.) I will not engage here in further lengthy discussion of conditions or criteria necessary for morally appropriate research involving healthy children. Instead I will simply offer the following suggested guidelines – all of which follow, I believe, from what I have said thus far:

(1) The experimental protocol should be meticulous in its formulation and should be subjected to institutional peer review.
(2) The experiment should offer a very real prospect of significant and essential new knowledge.
(3) The experiment must be a last resort – i.e., knowledge to be gained must be such that experimentation involving children is the only available means of attaining it. Where possible, the same or similiar experiment must have been conducted with adult subjects and been found to be without risk to them.
(4) An IRB must determine that the protocol involves no discernible risk or significant discomfort for children – nothing that children of that age would probably find painful or otherwise threatening.
(5) Parents should be given a detailed explanation of the protocol's purposes, procedures, and any known side-effects their children may experience. They should then verify that, as far as they know, their particular children would not be pained or frightened by those procedures or possible side-effects.
(6) Also, parents should express their own interest in the protocol's purposes by participating in it as co-subjects (where possible) or in some supervisory role.
(7) Children old enough to understand should be given a reasonably detailed description (on their level) of what their participation involves. This should be done not only by the researchers but also by an independent

subject-representative, perhaps a child psychologist. If they then choose not to participate, their dissents should be respected.

(8) Child-subjects who begin to exhibit significant anxiety or discomfort during the course of an experiment should be withdrawn from participation in it.

(9) Children who are mentally retarded and/or institutionalized should not be included as subjects. As McCormick has noted, the possibilities for experimental abuses are greater in their case than in the case of "normal" children living in families. Moreover, we have little reason to suspect that they will ever understand and accept many of the interests that their parents may presume on their behalf.

(10) A report of the protocol's findings and research significance should be sent to all subjects after the experiment's completion.[20]

Finally, I would offer a suggestion about the matter of "compensation" for children's nontherapeutic research participation. Healthy adult research "volunteers" are generally paid something for their participation. Such payments are not intended as "bribes" or coercions, although some potential subjects may view them in that way. (Indeed, IRB's are frequently faced with the difficult task of determining what level of payment is "reasonable" and commensurate with work-time lost and any potential discomforts, yet is also non-coercive.) The central moral purpose of such payments is to express the community's gratitude to those who have furthered the promise of medical advancement. So I would suggest that if adult subjects are 'thanked' in this way, then pediatric subjects should be, too. Perhaps the best form for this would be to give the parents a savings bond in the child's name, redeemable by the child-subject in the future. (Payments to parents who are co-subjects should not exceed the child's bond amount except perhaps to compensate for travel expenses and/or lost wages; and parents involved in a merely supervisory role should be compensated only for the latter purposes.) It should go without saying that this approach has the added advantage of providing another curb against abuses of proxy consent by parents who may be seeking their own (financial) interests rather than their children's presumed or explicit interests.[21]

Now, like the other two concrete moral issues examined above, the matter of nontherapeutic pediatric experimentation does not admit any easy answers. We face difficulties and ambiguities at every turn. But I have suggested here that *if* we have an interest in responding gratefully to the covenant invitation established by past research subjects; if we believe, hope, and expect that our children will share in that interest; and if we also remain committed to avoiding risk or discomfort for our children; then I believe there may be good moral grounds for allowing some (limited) nontherapeutic research with children.

SOME REFLECTIONS AND SUGGESTIONS 199

5. A POSTSCRIPT

The reflections offered in this chapter are not particularly ground-breaking or novel. Nor should they be seen as my attempt to provide the 'final word' in these difficult areas of medico-moral judgement. My hope is that they can be useful contributions to the ongoing theological-ethical dialogues in contemporary biomedicine – dialogues advanced so ably by McCormick, Ramsey, Hauerwas and Gustafson. For, as I have said before, it is through such dialogue that we can enlarge our own perspectives and make headway in our common quest for moral wisdom. Each of us comes to that task with somewhat different presuppositions, hopes, fears, and experiences; and exploration and analysis of those differences is a vehicle for our moral and spiritual growth. At the same time, of course, such exploration and analysis also leads to fuller discovery of the many perspectives, insights, and experiences we may share – even though we have expressed them in different terms. Finally, then, as James Gustafson has reminded us, "[t]he best one can expect to do is speak honestly for oneself, with some confidence that one's own experience is not utterly unique but similar to that of a significant number of persons" ([8], p. 759). That is what I have tried to do in the foregoing commentary, just as I believe it is what the four subjects of this study have been doing all along.

NOTES

[1] I realize that biblical claims about God's covenant promise – such as Paul's, cited here – might be viewed with some skepticism from within Gustafson's perspective. For, such expressions might be seen as scientifically insupportable, as "anthropocentric" in their import, or as insufficiently validated in the experience of contemporary persons. It is true, of course, that a 'sense' of God's unfailing, abiding love cannot be verified scientifically; but neither can it be disproven or shown to be misdirected. Further, that sense is not a sense of God's loving promise to me alone, or to human beings alone (e.g., Pauline theology expresses a sense of divine redemptive purpose inclusive of "all things" in creation [Col. 1:15–20]). Nor is it a sense that what I have previously experienced as good-for-me will always define the content and expression of what God's "love" toward me (or anyone or anything else) means. It is rather a sense that the Creator's own definition of "love" toward the created is fitting, and that, however I might experience that love, I will not be abandoned by the One who promises. Finally, with respect to experiential confirmation of claims such as Paul's, I would point out that while human experience of a sense of God's covenant promise has not been universal, it is an affective experience confirmed by many in the history of Christianity, and is confirmed again and again in the experiences of myself and the community of faith of which I am a part. And that is the only experience from which I can speak.

[2] It is worth noting here that in the Johannine version of Jesus's most famous depiction of the moral meaning of covenant response – his "love commandment" – his language is not abstract-propositional but rather the language of experiential analogy. The object of that analogy is, of course, the disciples' experience of Jesus himself. His moral imperative ("love one another") is qualified by analogy to his own life's indicative: *"as I have loved you"* (Jn. 13:34; 15:12).

[3] A recurring critique of many Catholic natural law approaches is that their definitions of 'the

good' (and how best to pursue those goods) appear a-historical and abstracted from the experience of 'good' in many persons' lives. Yet the approach taken by McCormick, the Catholic natural law theorist considered here, represents a clear attempt to bring traditional formulations into constructive dialogue with "human experience broadly conceived." Lisa Cahill comments, for example, that McCormick's "greatest contribution" to the natural law method "is to tie it more realistically to human experience and to individual and communal discretion" ([5], p. 101f.).

[4] McCormick's appeals to the divine gift of life were left unattended in Chapter 2 because of his more consistent focus upon life as a "relative good." However, his corpus does include such explicit claims as: "Thus life is a gift, a trust. It has great worth because of the value He is placing in it . . ." ([14], p. 30).

[5] In contrast, return of a gift based upon the recipient's express desire to insult the donor or to show contempt for the gift (or of others who value it) would be seen as morally offensive.

[6] In other words, I cannot accept Gustafson's clean and simple solution to the traditional problem of *theodicy*. And, as Margaret Pabst Battin reminds us, "the answer to the overriding question of whether gratitude to God [for the 'gift' of life] is appropriate or morally required, even when the life He has bestowed is unsatisfactory, depends on the type of theodicy we employ" ([2], p. 45).

[7] See, e.g., [9], pp. 153–54.

[8] David Rivlin died, in the manner he chose, in a friend's home on July 20, 1989 [26]. He was offered the assistance of Dr. Jack Kevorkian and his "suicide machine," but refused that route. Finally, he was aided by a local hospice physician who administered the necessary sedation prior to removal of the respirator.

[9] In the Hebrew Scriptures, Abimelech, Samson, Saul and his armor-bearer, Ahitophel, and Zimri; in the Apocrypha, Razis and Ptolemy Macron; and in the New Testament, Judas (see [2], pp. 29–38).

[10] For example, decisions for death-by-nontreatment in order to express contempt for family members or caregivers, or when one is still able to provide material and/or psychic support for one's dependents without significantly increased suffering for oneself represent, in my view, failures of moral obligation.

[11] For brevity's sake I am not dealing here with several important (and complicating) matters – among them the question of how we determine a patient's basic *competence* to make decisions of this sort, and the matter of specific patient expectations (of prognosis or future incapacity) which appear clinically unreasonable or 'delusional.' I am presuming, for purposes of this discussion, the existence of patients whose general competence and comprehension (of available clinical predictions in their cases) are not in question.

[12] This case is adapted from [15] and [17].

[13] The practical cloudiness of such diagnostic/prognostic distinctions is illustrated graphically in Peggy and Robert Stinson's memoir of their son Andrew's treatment and eventual death, entitled *The Long Dying of Baby Andrew* [24].

[14] At least one judicial decision has held that infant patients in persistent vegetative states do not fit the precise technical definition of "chronic and irreversible coma" as included in the federal statute's wording. But pediatric specialists have argued that persistent vegetative state must be the real referent of the statutory exception, since children do not remain "chronically and irreversibly comatose" for long. (See, e.g., [3].)

[15] My reflections here omit any reference to purely "vitalistic" approaches to assessing an infant's best interests, in part because such an approach is not advocated by any of the moralists surveyed here, but primarily because I agree with McCormick's assertion that such approaches have no reasonable grounding in Christian Scripture and/or tradition.

[16] Ramsey and McCormick agree that infants facing intractable pain – pain that would overwhelm their reception of care and human presence or inhibit their relational potential – have little interest in prolonged life. Hauerwas's critique of our "Promethean" attempts to eliminate suf-

fering (even to the point of eliminating the sufferer) leads me to wonder whether he would agree fully with them in this regard. On the other hand, Hauerwas is also critical of "heroic" prolongation of infants' lives in order to make us feel better about ourselves, since that could lead us to subject retarded children to "forms of care that they should not be forced to undergo." The obvious inference here is that life-prolonging treatment clearly is not in some infants' best interests; and infants in chronic and severe pain (or treatments which will cause them such pain) may be among the examples Hauerwas has in mind.

[17] Feeding is certainly a part of "comfort care" in most instances. But I agree with McCormick and Paris that it may be considered morally optional in some cases (e.g., of severe necrotizing enterocolitis or short-bowel syndrome) where it can only be provided artificially, cannot sustain life for very long, and is itself a source of discomfort. Analgesia (for whatever discomfort starvation/dehydration may being) is especially important in such cases.

[18] See, for example, [25] – esp. Chapter 9.

[19] See, for example, [11].

[20] Conditions 1–4 are adapted from Bartholome's list of guidelines in [1], p. 3.20.

[21] I will not deal here with another issue of research "compensation" – namely, appropriate compensation for persons who are accidentally injured as a result of their research participation.

REFERENCES

1. Bartholome, W.: 1977, 'The Ethics of Non-Therapeutic Clinical Research on Children', in the National Commission for the Protection of Human Subjects of Biomedical and Behavioral Research, *Research Involving Children: APPENDIX*, DHEW Publication No. (OS)77–000s, Washington, D.C., pp. 3.1–3.22.
2. Battin, M.P.: 1982, *Ethical Issues in Suicide*, Prentice-Hall, Englewood Cliffs, N.J.
3. Bermel, J.: 1986, 'Confusion Over the Language of the Baby Doe Regulations', *Hastings Center Report* 16/6, 2.
4. Bonhoeffer, D.: 1955, *Ethics* (trans. and ed. by E. Bethge), Macmillan, New York.
5. Cahill, L.: 1993, 'On Richard McCormick: Reason and Faith in Post-Vatican II Catholic Ethics', in A. Verhey and S. Lammers (eds.), *Theological Voices in Medical Ethics*, Eerdmans, Grand Rapids, pp. 78–105.
6. Camenisch, P.: 1981, 'Gift and Gratitude in Ethics', *Journal of Religious Ethics* 9/1, 1–34.
7. Gustafson, J.: 1978, *Protestant and Roman Catholic Ethics: Prospects for Rapprochement*, University of Chicago Press, Chicago.
8. Gustafson, J.: 1980, 'A Theocentric Interpretation of Life', *The Christian Century* 97, 754–760.
9. Hauerwas, S.: 1977, *Truthfulness and Tragedy: Further Explorations Into Christian Ethics*, University of Notre Dame Press, Notre Dame.
10. Hauerwas, S.: 1986, *Suffering Presence: Theological Reflections on Medicine, the Mentally Handicapped, and the Church*, University of Notre Dame Press, Notre Dame.
11. Ingelfinger, F.: 1972, 'Informed (But Uneducated) Consent', *New England Journal of Medicine* 287/9, 465–466.
12. Jonas, H.: 1970, 'Philosophical Reflections on Experimenting With Human Subjects', in P. Freund (ed.), *Experimentation With Human Subjects*, George Braziller, Inc., New York, pp. 1–31.
13. Kluge, E-H.: 1975, *The Practice of Death*, Yale University Press, New Haven.
14. McCormick, R.: 1982, 'Theology and Biomedical Ethics', *Logos* 3, 25–45.
15. 'Man Freed in Comatose Son's Death': 1989, *Detroit Free Press*, May 19, 1A–2A.
16. May, W.: 1983, *The Physician's Covenant: Images of the Healer in Medical Ethics*, Westminster, Philadelphia.

17. Miles, S.: 1989, 'Taking Hostages: The Linares Case', *Hastings Center Report* 19/4, 4.
18. Miles, S. et al.: 1989, 'Conflicts Between Patients' Wishes to Forgo Treatment and the Policies of Health Care Facilities', *New England Journal of Medicine* 321/1, 48–50.
19. Ramsey, P.: 1950, *Basic Christian Ethics*, Charles Scribners Sons, New York.
20. Ramsey, P.: 1962, *Nine Modern Moralists*, Prentice-Hall, Engelwood Cliffs, N.J.
21. Ramsey, P.: 1967, *Deeds and Rules in Christian Ethics*, Charles Scribners Sons, New York.
22. Ramsey, P.: 1970, *The Patient as Person*, Yale University Press, New Haven.
23. Ross, W.D.: 1939, *The Foundations of Ethics*, Clarendon Press, Oxford.
24. Stinson, R. and Stinson, P.: 1983, *The Long Dying of Baby Andrew*, Atlantic Monthly Press, New York.
25. Weir, R.: 1984, *Selective Nontreatment of Handicapped Newborns*, Oxford University Press, New York.
26. Williams, M.: 1989, 'An End to Emptiness', *Detroit Free Press*, July 21, 1A, 15A.
27. Williams, M.: 1989, 'Paralyzed 18 Years, Man Asks Court to Let Him End Life', *Detroit Free Press*, May 19, 1A–2A.

INDEX

Abimelech 200n.
abortion 22, 25, 45, 92n., 127n.
affectivity, religious 134–37
agape, 2, 3, 55–65, 92n., 97, 146, 156
"agapism" 61ff., 89
Ahitophel 200n.
Albrecht, Gloria 108f., 126n.
allocation (of health care costs) 187–89
American Medical Association 15
Anscombe, G.E.M. 40f., 42
anthropocentrism 132f., 138, 143, 157, 161, 199n.
Aquinas, Thomas 1, 13f., 37f., 48n., 50n., 90n., 143, 148–49
Aristotle 37
Arras, John D. 49n.
artificial insemination 88
Augustine 140, 179

"Baby Doe" case (1992) 5, 68, 120, 151
Baier, Kurt 50n.
Barth, Karl 57, 60, 147f.
Bartholome, William 194ff., 201n.
Battin, Margaret Pabst 93n., 200n.
beatitudo 37, 143, 158
Bentham, Jeremy 39, 41
Bergmeier, Mrs. (case) 26, 64
Bok, Sissela 187
Boley, William 160, 162n.
bombing, obliteration 26f., 42, 65
Bondi, Richard 112f.
Bonhoeffer, Dietrich 169ff., 177
bonum honestum 18
bonum utile 18, 31
Bouvia, Elizabeth (case) 8, 77, 178
Broad, C.D. 36
Burrell, David 127n.

Cahill, Lisa 36, 45, 48, 50n., 90, 92n., 200n.
"Caiaphas principle" 25
Camenisch, Paul 91n., 173ff.
Campbell, A.G.M. 4
Carney, Frederick 35
character 98–109

Child Abuse Amendments of 1984 5f., 92n., 180f., 186f., 200n.
children,
  attitudes toward 116–21
  research involving 9ff., 31–35, 81–89, 121–26, 155–60, 190–98
  rights of 123f.
Childress, James F. 36, 47, 61, 77, 93n., 160, 162n.
Christian ethics, distinctiveness of 19f., 59f., 97, 106–109, 130f., 138, 167–72
Christology 138f.
Church, identity of 106–109
compensation (for research participation) 198, 201n.
Connery, John 35f., 38, 80, 93n.
Conroy case (New Jersey) 5
conscientious objection 186
consequentialism 35–48, 50n., 56, 103, 122, 160, 165
"Constantinianism" 107
contraception 1, 23,
Copleston, F.C. 50n.
covenant fidelity 3, 55–65, 81–89, 90n., 92n., 122, 146, 156, 165, 170f., 190
covenant promise 168–72, 176, 188, 199n.
covenant-response, ethic of 168–72, 177, 190ff.
Cruzan case 7
Curran, Charles 1, 47, 58

death, theological meaning of 15f., 66–68, 91n., 92n., 110f., 113–16, 118, 147f.
deontology 23, 36f., 50n., 55, 62f., 96, 122, 141, 166, 170
determinism,
  social 99
  divine 138
discernment, theocentric 140–46
discrimen 164
double effect, principle of 21ff., 42'
draft, military 35, 157f.
Duff, Raymond 5
Dunlop, Sir Derrick 61

203

INDEX

Edwards, Jonathan 140
equity 58
euthanasia, active 42, 69ff., 75f., 78–81, 92n., 112f., 127n.
evangelism 168f.
Evans, Donald 42, 91n.
evil, "physical" ("premoral") and moral 22ff., 38, 44, 49n.
exceptions (to moral rules) 61–65, 91n., 170

family, meaning of 123f., 152f., 185f., 187f.
Feinberg, Joel 49n., 93n.
Finnis, John 43f.
Fletcher, Joseph 26, 41, 54, 91n.
Frankena, William 36, 61f.
freedom 26f., 29, 57, 61, 63, 76, 79, 100, 105f., 112–15, 117, 126n., 127n., 179, 191
Fuchs, Joseph 49n.
"fundamental requisites" 143f.

gift,
    children as 116f., 176
    death as 66, 111
    definition of 80f., 93n.
    life as 76, 79–81, 110f., 147f., 150f., 172–80, 200n.
Giraudoux, Jean 126n.
God, glorification of 158f.
Golden Rule 183
gratitude (as ground of Christian ethics) 168–72, 191f.
Grisez, Germain 35, 44
Gustafson, James M. 4, 107, 130–63, 164ff., 167f., 169, 175f., 182, 190, 199, 200n.

Hare, R.M. 51n.
Harris, Charles 92n.
Hauerwas, Stanley 4, 86–129, 131, 142, 148, 150, 154, 162n., 165f., 176f., 182, 184, 187f., 193f., 200n.
Humanae vitae, 1

inclinationes naturales 19
infants, treatment decisions for 5, 14–19, 65–74, 116–21, 151–55, 180–89
Institutional Ethics Committee 180, 186f.
Institutional Review Board 196f.
integrity 96

interactional model (of human agency) 140, 144–46, 150
intuitionism 57

Janssens, Louis 49n.
Jehovah's Witnesses 11n.
"Johns Hopkins case" 5, 119, 151–55
Johnson, Mark 93n.
Jonas, Hans 84, 191f.

Kant, Immanuel 85, 104, 113, 122, 148–49, 162n.
Kelly, Gerald 15
Kevorkian, Jack 200n.
Kluge, Eike–Henner 174f.
Knauer, Peter 38f.

Lakoff, George 93n.
Langan, John 50n., 51n.
Lehmann, Paul 54, 91n.
Lesch–Nyhan Syndrome 71ff., 185
liberalism 105f., 126n.
Linares, Samuel (case) 180f., 187, 189
listening, ethic of 171
Luther, Martin 57

McClendon, James 108
McCormick, Richard A. 3, 13–53, 55, 65f., 68, 74, 82–84, 88ff., 92n., 97, 119, 124f., 147, 150, 154, 158–60, 164ff., 179, 182ff., 192f., 194, 198, 200n., 201n.
MacIntyre, Alasdair 36, 122
McKenny, Gerald 131
macroallocation 166
Maritain, Jacques 59
Marty, Martin 107
masturbation 23, 38, 49n., 50n.
May, William F. 90n., 168
Mead, G.H. 99, 126n.
"medical indications policy" (Ramsey) 68–81, 121, 127n., 181ff.
metaphor 80f., 93n.
middle axioms 19, 47
Mill, J.S. 39, 148
Milton, John 161
Moore, G.E. 40
Murdoch, Iris 100

narratives 98, 101–109, 131, 176f.
Natanson v. *Kline* 7

natural law 1, 13f., 19, 37f., 48, 49n., 50n., 56f., 59, 61, 124, 137, 142, 146, 158, 164, 199n., 200n.
necessity, criterion of (McCormick) 24ff., 43, 45, 48
Niebuhr, H. Richard 107
Niebuhr, Reinhold 54
non-violence 104f., 126n.

O'Connell, Timothy 13f.
order 58f.
'ordinary'/'extraordinary' means of treatment 14ff., 74–77, 93n., 127n., 153, 162n.
ordo bonorum 21, 26ff., 30, 47f., 97, 154, 158
Outka, Gene 91n., 99

Paris, John 17f., 201n.
participation (in the divine ordering) 140–46
parts (and wholes) 144–46, 150, 155, 157–61
paternalism 28f., 115, 145, 180, 194
Patient Self-Determination Act 7
Paul (apostle) 66, 111, 168, 199n.
Paul VI 1, 49n.
piety 4, 134f., 136–39
Pius XII 16
polis 122
"preference principles" (McCormick) 20f.
prima facie duties 23
primum non nocere ("first, do no harm") 12n., 84, 156, 157
property-rights 58
proportionate reason 21ff., 30f., 35–48, 66
Ptolemy Macron 200n.

quality of life 6, 16ff., 65–74, 93n., 153f., 181–84
Quinlan, Karen Ann 70f.

Ramsey, Paul 3, 34, 51n., 54–93, 97, 115, 121–22, 127n., 147f., 150, 156f., 162n., 165f., 170f., 174f. 181ff., 190–95, 200n.
rape 65
Rawls, John 91n.
Razis 200n.
Reeder, John P. 143f.
Reformed theology 136f.
Reich, Warren 73
Reiner, Hans 20

relational potential 16ff., 49n., 119, 154, 182ff.
relativism 97, 101f., 144
research (medical),
   'gifts' of 191f.
   imperative of 12, 84, 87, 147
   nontherapeutic pediatric 9ff., 31–35, 46, 81–89, 121–26, 155–60, 190–98
rights, positive and negative 78f., 93n.
Rivlin, David (case) 178f., 200n.
Robinson, John A.T. 54, 91n.
Rosebush case (Michigan) 6
Ross, W.D. 23, 36f., 41, 166

Salk, Jonas 82
Samson 179, 200n.
sanctity of life 6f., 17f., 66–68, 78, 92n., 110
Saul, King 179, 200n.
Schenck, David 161n.
Schuller, Bruno 23, 49n.
science, as test of theological assertions 136ff., 145
Scripture, interpretation of 108f.
self, agency of 98–103, 112–15, 150
self-deception 100, 120, 176
Sidgewick, Henry 148
sin, restraint of 58f., 88f., 90n.
"slippery slope" 79, 86
Singer, Peter 45, 51n.
sociality 33, 35, 159, 192f.
Speer, Albert 127n.
sterilization, contraceptive 23, 38, 65
stewardship 140
Stinson, Peggy and Robert 200n.
strangers, children as 120, 123
substituted judgement 32, 34, 83
suffering, interpretation of 114f., 117f., 123, 127n., 154
suicide 14, 29, 77–81, 93n., 110, 112f., 114f., 148–51, 175, 179
"summary rules" 63
Summa Theologiae 1, 13, 37
summum bonum 45, 47, 56, 6

Tay–Sachs Disease 72f., 185
teleology 19ff., 35–39, 55f., 62f., 96, 143, 164, 166
"theocentrism," defined 132f.
theodicy 133, 200n.
Tillich, Paul 138

tragedy 103, 111f.
tragic choices 86
treatment, refusal of 7–9, 28–31, 74–81, 93n., 110–16, 146–51, 172–80
Troeltsch, Ernst 136

"unconsented touching," injury of 85
utilitarianism 35ff., 39–48, 50n., 127n., 141, 160, 196

Veatch, Robert 49n., 127n.

vision 98–109, 140
Visscher, Maurice 12n.

Walzer, Michael 86f.
wedge argument 79, 86, 93n.
Willimon, William 108

Yoder, John H. 108

Zimri 200n.

Theology and Medicine

Managing Editor

Earl E. Shelp, *The Foundation for Interfaith Research & Ministry, Houston, Texas*

1. R.M. Green (ed.): *Religion and Sexual Health.* Ethical, Theological and Clinical Perspectives. 1992 ISBN 0-7923-1752-1
2. P.F. Camenisch (ed.): *Religious Methods and Resources in Bioethics.* 1994
ISBN 0-7923-2102-2
3. G.M. McKenney and J.R. Sande (eds.): *Theological Analyses of the Clinical Encounter.* 1994 ISBN 0-7923-2362-9
4. C.S. Campbell and B.A. Lustig (eds.): *Duties to Others.* 1994 ISBN 0-7923-2638-5
5. E.R. DuBose: *The Illusion of Trust.* Toward a Medical Theological Ethics in the Postmodern Age. 1995 ISBN 0-7923-3144-3
6. L.S. Cahill and M.A. Farley (eds.): *Embodiment, Morality, and Medicine.* 1995
ISBN 0-7923-3342-X
7. J.B. Tubbs, Jr.: *Christian Theology and Medical Ethics.* Four Contemporary Approaches. 1996 ISBN 0-7923-3657-7

KLUWER ACADEMIC PUBLISHERS – DORDRECHT / BOSTON / LONDON